THE ESSENTIAL FERTILITY FOOD COOKBOOK

A Culinary Guide to Optimal Reproductive Wellness:Nourishing Recipes for Your Path to Parenthood"

Bonus: 30 days meal plan for you

By
Peggy M. Tharp

Copyright

Disclaimer

The information provided in this Essential Fertility Food cook book is for general informational purposes only. It is not intended as medical, health or nutritional advice and should not be construed as such. The content is based on the author's personal experiences, research, and knowledge as of the date of publication.

Readers are advised to consult with qualified healthcare professionals for individualized advice regarding their specific health or medical conditions. The author and publisher disclaim any liability for any adverse effects resulting directly or indirectly from the use or application of the information contained in this Essential Fertility Food Cookbook

While every effort has been made to ensure the accuracy and completeness of the information provided, the author and publisher assume no responsibility for errors, inaccuracies, omissions, or any inconsistencies herein. Any reliance on the information in this Essential Fertility Food cookbook is at the reader's own risk.

About the author

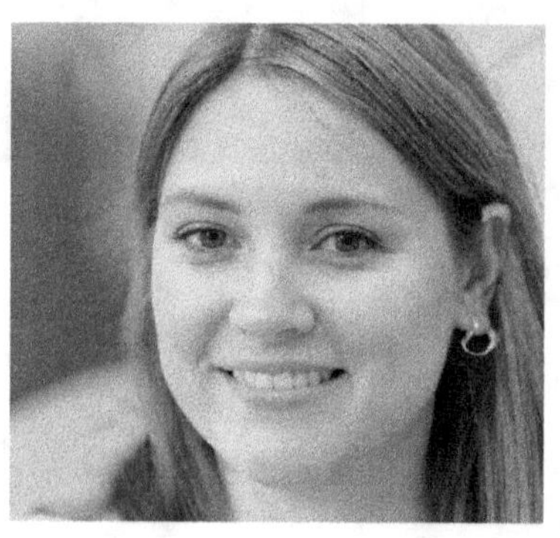

Meet Peggy M. Tharp,a dedicated and passionate fertility expert in the realm of nutrition and food. With a profound interest in the intersection of fertility and culinary arts, Peggy M. Tharp has devoted her expertise to crafting nourishing recipes that support reproductive health.

Drawing from a background rooted in nutrition and a deep understanding of the intricate relationship between food and fertility, Peggy M. Tharp brings a unique perspective to the world of fertility cookbooks. Her commitment to empowering individuals on their journey to parenthood is reflected in the thoughtfully curated recipes designed to enhance fertility and overall well-being.

Peggy M. Tharp believes in the transformative power of food, recognizing it not only as sustenance but as a powerful ally in the pursuit of optimal reproductive health. Her culinary creations are a testament to the idea that embracing fertility-focused nutrition can be both delicious and rewarding.

In addition to her expertise in fertility-enhancing foods, Peggy M. Tharp is an avid writer who finds joy in sharing her knowledge with a wider audience. Her passion for educating and guiding individuals on the path to parenthood has led her to embark on the journey of writing fertility cookbooks. Through her books, Peggy M. Tharp aims to provide accessible and practical insights into the world of fertility-friendly cooking.

Whether you are starting your fertility journey or seeking to optimize your reproductive health, Peggy M. Tharp invites you to explore the transformative potential of embracing fertility-focused cuisine. With a blend of expertise, creativity, and a genuine desire to make a positive impact, Peggy M. Tharp is committed to helping individuals nourish their bodies and embark on the rewarding path towards parenthood through the art of food.

Bonus: 30 days meal plan

DAY 1:

Breakfast: Greek yogurt with mixed berries and pumpkin seeds

Snack: Carrot sticks with hummus or sunflower seeds

Lunch: Quinoa salad with chickpeas, roasted vegetables, and lemon vinaigrette

Snack: Apple slices with almond butter

Dinner: Salmon with roasted asparagus and sweet potato

DAY 2:

Breakfast: Smoothie with spinach, banana, and almond milk

Snack: Trail mix with nuts, seeds, and dried fruit

Lunch: Lentil soup with whole-wheat bread

Snack: Edamame with sea salt

Dinner: Chicken stir-fry with brown rice and broccoli

DAY 3:

Breakfast: Whole-wheat toast with avocado and eggs

Snack: Berries with Greek yogurt

Lunch: Tuna salad sandwich on whole-wheat bread

Snack: Roasted chickpeas with spices

Dinner: Lentil pasta with marinara sauce and vegetables

DAY 4

Breakfast: Oatmeal with nuts and seeds

Snack: Cottage cheese with pineapple

Lunch: Chicken Caesar salad with whole-wheat croutons

Snack: Dark chocolate-covered almonds

Dinner: Shrimp scampi with whole-wheat pasta and zucchini noodles

DAY 5

Breakfast: Chia pudding with almond milk and fruit

Snack: Apple slices with peanut butter

Black bean burgers on whole-wheat buns with sweet potato chips for lunch

Snack: Hummus with whole-wheat pita bread

Dinner: Tofu stir-fry with quinoa and vegetables

DAY 6

Breakfast: Scrambled eggs with spinach and whole-wheat toast

Snack: Carrot sticks with guacamole

Lunch: Leftovers from the week

Snack: Hard-boiled eggs

Dinner: Turkey chili with brown rice and avocado

DAY 7

Breakfast: Smoothie with kale, mango, and almond milk

Snack: Blueberries with almonds

Lunch: Tuna salad with avocado on whole-wheat crackers

Snack: Trail mix with nuts, seeds, and dried fruit

Dinner: Baked cod with roasted root vegetables

DAY 8

Breakfast: Whole-wheat pancakes with berries and nuts

Snack: Roasted pumpkin seeds with cinnamon

Lunch: Black bean and corn salad with salsa and tortilla chips

Snack: Cottage cheese with pineapple and chia seeds

Dinner: Veggie burgers on whole-wheat buns with grilled onions and sweet potato fries

DAY 9

Breakfast: Omelet with mushrooms and bell peppers

Snack: Apple slices with almond butter and cinnamon

Lunch: grilled chicken salad with mixed vegetables and quinoa

Snack: Greek yogurt with honey and granola

Dinner: Vegetarian lasagna with ricotta and Spinach

DAY 10

Breakfast: Greek yogurt with fruit and granola

Snack: Trail mix with nuts, seeds, and dried fruit

Lunch: Leftovers from the week

Snack: Edamame with sea salt and lime juice

Dinner: roasted Brussels sprouts and quinoa with salmon

DAY 11

Breakfast: Chia seed overnight oats with almond milk

Snack: Cottage cheese with pineapple and mango

Lunch: Lentil and vegetable soup with whole-grain bread

Snack: Hummus on whole-wheat pita bread with cucumber slices

Dinner: Vegetarian stew with crusty bread

DAY 12

Breakfast: Whole-wheat waffles with berries and nut butter

Snack: roasted chickpeas with paprika and garlic spice

Lunch: Leftovers from the week

Snack: Dark chocolate with fruits

Dinner: Chicken pot pie with whole-wheat biscuits

DAY 13

Breakfast: Kale, banana, and almond milk smoothie

Snack: Trail mix with nuts, seeds, and dried fruit

Lunch: lentil and vegetable curry over brown rice

Snack: Greek yogurt with honey and granola

Dinner: Turkey chili with cornbread

DAY 14

Breakfast: Eggs Benedict with whole-wheat English muffins

Snack: Carrot sticks with guacamole

Lunch: Leftovers from the week

Snack: Hard-boiled eggs with avocado toast

Dinner: Salmon with roasted vegetables and couscous

DAY 15

Breakfast: Whole-wheat pancakes with ricotta and peaches

Snack: Mixed nuts and dried fruit

Lunch: Tuna salad sandwich on whole-wheat bread with avocado

Snack: Greek yogurt with berries and chia seeds

Dinner: Chicken fajitas with whole-wheat tortillas and roasted vegetables

DAY 16

Breakfast: Spinach, feta cheese, and tomatoes omelet

Snack: Apple slices with almond butter

Lunch: Leftovers from the week

Snack: Edamame with sea salt

Dinner: Black bean soup with whole-grain tortillas and avocado

DAY 17

Breakfast: Fruit salad with yogurt and granola

Snack: Cottage cheese with pineapple

Lunch: Lentil and vegetable salad with balsamic vinaigrette

Snack: Trail mix with nuts, seeds, and dried fruit

Dinner: Shrimp scampi with whole-wheat pasta and roasted tomatoes

DAY 18

Breakfast: Smoothie with spinach, mango, and coconut water

Snack: Roasted chickpeas with spices

Lunch: Chicken Caesar salad with homemade dressing

Snack: Hummus with whole-wheat pita bread

Dinner: Salmon with roasted fennel and lemon sauce

DAY 19

Breakfast: Whole-wheat waffles with Greek yogurt and honey

Snack: Dark chocolate with fruits

Lunch: Leftovers from the week

Snack: Hard-boiled eggs

Dinner: Lentil Shepherd's pie with cauliflower mash

DAY 20

Breakfast: Scrambled eggs with chives and smoked salmon

Snack: Carrot sticks with guacamole

Lunch: grilled chicken wrap with hummus and veggies

Snack: Yogurt with granola and pumpkin seeds

Dinner: Chicken cacciatore with whole-wheat pasta and green beans

DAY 21

Breakfast: Kale, banana, and almond milk smoothie

Snack: Blueberries with almonds

Lunch: Quinoa salad with chickpeas, roasted vegetables, and lemon vinaigrette

Snack: Dark chocolate-covered almonds

Dinner: Salmon with roasted asparagus and sweet potato

DAY 22

Breakfast: Chia seed overnight oats with almond milk

Snack: Apple slices with peanut butter

Lunch: Lentil and vegetable soup with whole-grain bread

Snack: Roasted chickpeas with spices

Dinner: Chicken stir-fry with brown rice and broccoli

DAY 23

Breakfast: Whole-wheat toast with avocado and eggs

Snack: Berries with Greek yogurt

Lunch: Tuna salad sandwich on whole-wheat bread

Snack: Trail mix with nuts, seeds, and dried fruit

Dinner: Lentil pasta with marinara sauce and vegetables

DAY 24

Breakfast: Oatmeal with nuts and seeds

Snack: Edamame with sea salt

Lunch: Chicken Caesar salad with whole-wheat croutons

Snack: Cottage cheese with pineapple

Dinner: Shrimp scampi with whole-wheat pasta and zucchini noodles

DAY 25

Breakfast: Chia pudding with almond milk and fruit

Snack: Roasted chickpeas with spices

Lunch: Black bean burgers on whole-wheat buns with sweet potato fries

Snack: Dark chocolate with fruits

Dinner: Tofu stir-fry with quinoa and vegetables

DAY 26

Breakfast: Scrambled eggs with spinach and whole-wheat toast

Snack: Carrot sticks with guacamole

Lunch: Leftovers from the week

Snack: Hummus with whole-wheat pita bread

Dinner: Turkey chili over brown rice with avocado.

DAY 27

Breakfast: Smoothie with kale, mango, and almond milk

Snack: Trail mix with nuts, seeds, and dried fruit

Lunch: Tuna salad with avocado on whole-wheat crackers

Snack: Hard-boiled eggs

Dinner: Baked cod with roasted root vegetables

DAY 28

Breakfast: Kale, banana, and almond milk smoothie

Snack: Berries with Greek yogurt and hemp seeds

Lunch: Quinoa salad with chickpeas, roasted vegetables, and lemon vinaigrette

Snack: Dark chocolate-covered almonds

Dinner: Salmon with roasted asparagus and sweet potato

DAY 29

Breakfast: Chia seed overnight oats with almond milk

Snack: Peanut butter and cinnamon-topped sliced apples

Lunch: Lentil and vegetable soup with whole-grain bread

Snack: Roasted chickpeas with spices

Dinner: Chicken stir-fry with brown rice and broccoli

DAY 30

Breakfast: Whole-wheat toast with avocado and eggs

Snack: Trail mix with nuts, seeds, and dried fruit

Lunch: Tuna salad sandwich on whole-wheat bread

Snack: Cucumber slices and whole-wheat pita bread with hummus.

Dinner: Lentil pasta with marinara sauce and vegetables

Table of contents

INTRODUCTION

Welcome to "Prolific Blowouts: Feeding Your Excursion to Being a parent." This cookbook is something other than an assortment of recipes; it's an aid intended to help and improve your richness through the influence of healthy, supporting food varieties. In the pages that follow, you'll find a culinary excursion custom-made to advance your wellbeing as well as your general health as you explore the way to parenthood. Our painstakingly created recipes center around the standards of wellbeing, equilibrium, and richness cordial nourishment. Each dish is nicely ready to give fundamental supplements, nutrients, and minerals known to add to regenerative prosperity. From supplement rich morning meals to tasty suppers and liberal yet well being cognizant treats, these recipes are meant to motivate and sustain each step of your ripeness process.

All through this cookbook, you'll track down something beyond delectable recipes. We dive into the nourishing parts of each dish, offering experiences into key nutrients, planning tips, and serving ideas. As you investigate these pages, consider this a cookbook as well as a friend on your way to being a parent, giving you the devices and information to make informed, fruitfulness steady decisions in your day to day dinners.

Thus, whether you're simply starting your fruitfulness process or trying to improve your general prosperity, "Ripe Banquets" is here to direct you. Let the specialty of cooking become a wellspring of happiness and strengthening as you set out on this interesting part. May each chomp bring you fulfillment as well as a bit nearer to the health and life as a parent you want.

Let the excursion to richness and delightful living initiate!

Importance Of Fertility

The importance of nutrition in fertility cannot be overstated. It influences not only your ability to conceive but also the health and development of your potential child. Here's why:

For Women:

Egg Quality: Adequate intake of nutrients like folic acid, zinc, iron, and vitamins C and E helps in healthy egg development and maturation, increasing the chances of successful fertilization.

Hormonal Balance: Vitamins like D and B6 regulate hormones like estrogen and progesterone, crucial for ovulation and menstrual cycle regularity.

Endometrial Lining: Proper nutrition ensures a thick and healthy endometrial lining, vital for implantation and embryo growth.

Reduced Risk of Complications: A balanced diet reduces the risk of gestational diabetes, preeclampsia, and other pregnancy complications.

For Men:

Sperm Production and Quality: Zinc, selenium, vitamin C, and vitamin E are essential for healthy sperm production, motility, and morphology (shape), enhancing fertilization chances.

Hormonal Balance: Adequate zinc and vitamin D levels contribute to balanced testosterone levels, crucial for sperm production and male fertility.

Reduced DNA Damage: Antioxidants from fruits and vegetables protect sperm from oxidative damage, leading to healthier quality and reduced risk of miscarriage.

Overall Health:

Weight Management: Maintaining a healthy weight reduces risks associated with obesity, such as hormonal imbalances and ovulatory dysfunction, that can hinder fertility.

Energy Levels: A balanced diet provides sustained energy, critical for coping with the physical and emotional demands of pregnancy and parenthood.

Reduced Risk of Birth Defects: Adequate folic acid intake before and during pregnancy significantly reduces the risk of neural tube defects in babies.

Therefore, proper nutrition is not just an add-on for fertility; it's a foundation for creating a healthy environment for conception, pregnancy, and beyond. Focusing on a balanced diet rich in fruits, vegetables, whole grains, lean protein, and healthy fats provides the necessary nutrients for both partners to optimize their fertility potential.

Remember, consulting a healthcare professional or registered dietitian can help personalize your nutritional plan to address specific needs and boost your chances of a successful pregnancy journey.

How This Book Can Help You In Your Journey

Chasing being a parent, this cookbook arises as a directing buddy, offering something other than recipes. It turns into a guide, unpredictably intended to help and improve your excursion.

Inside these pages, every recipe is a cautiously organized commitment to your fruitfulness objectives. Past simple food, the culinary manifestations act as purposeful strides toward hormonal equilibrium, regenerative wellbeing, and the unpredictable dance of origination.

Think about this cookbook as a story unfurling on your plate. From dawn to nightfall, each dish is made with a guarantee to your special process, mixing every dinner with a hint of affection and a smidgen of pleasure.

Installed inside the recipes is an abundance of nourishing bits of knowledge. It's not just about the fixings; it's a potential chance to figure out the significant effect of explicit supplements on your fruitfulness goals. This information changes your dinners into deliberate demonstrations of taking care of oneself and sustenance.

Embrace the way of thinking of careful sustenance that pervades the cookbook. Each dinner is an event to intentionally interface with your body and yearnings. The flavors you enjoy reach out past taste, turning into a substantial articulation of your obligation to your richness process.

Inside these recipes lie the cell reinforcements, your partners against the tempests of oxidative pressure. Past their job as fixings, they stand monitor, safeguarding your contraceptive cells and establishing a climate helpful for your richness desires.

Consider this cookbook a material where you paint your culinary inclinations and richness goals. It welcomes you to try, investigate, and find an orchestra of tastes that reverberates with your extraordinary sense of taste and objectives.

This cookbook spans custom and science, offering a conversion of hereditary insight and present day nourishing experiences. An excursion traverses ages, mixing immortal culinary practices with the most recent comprehension of fruitfulness nourishment.

With each nibble, relish the commitment that you're supporting your body as well as a fruitful ground where the fantasies of life as a parent can flourish and prosper. This cookbook is in excess of an assortment of recipes; it's a murmured promise that each feast carries you nearer to the acknowledgment of your being a parent yearnings.

CHAPTER 1: FERTILITY BASICS

The fundamental ideas that guide the intricate process of conception and pregnancy are summed up in the term "fertility basics." At its center, this idea spins around understanding the physiological and organic factors that add to a couple's capacity to consider and effectively convey a pregnancy to term.

Integral to fruitfulness nuts and bolts is the monthly cycle, a musical ensemble of hormonal variances organizing the readiness of the female body for likely pregnancy. A crucial point in this cycle is when an egg is released from the ovary, which creates a limited window of opportunity for conception. Understanding the subtleties of this cycle is essential for couples to determine the best time to try to conceive.

Recognizing the significance of male reproductive factors in the process of conception, sperm health is another fundamental aspect of fertility basics. Within the fertility narrative, the journey of sperm from its production in the testes to its pursuit of the awaiting egg is a remarkable narrative. Factors, for example, sperm count, motility, and morphology are fundamental parts, affecting the probability of treatment

.Age arises as a basic consideration of fruitfulness essentials, especially for ladies. The biological fact of declining fertility with age emphasizes the significance of timely family planning. Decisions regarding the ideal time to start a family are informed by an understanding of how age affects reproductive capabilities.

In addition, basic fertility factors are heavily influenced by lifestyle choices. Reproductive health is influenced by diet, exercise, smoking, alcohol consumption, stress management, and other factors. A well-balanced and healthy lifestyle becomes a factor in fertility outcomes as well as a personal wellness choice.

Fundamentally, fruitfulness rudiments act as the compass directing couples through the complicated landscape of family arranging. They envelop the comprehension of contraceptive cycles, the meaning of the two accomplices' regenerative wellbeing, the effect old enough, and the job of way of life in molding fruitfulness results. Outfitted with this information, couples leave on their fruitfulness process with educated choices and a thorough comprehension regarding the natural embroidery that unfurls on their way to life as a parent.

Explaining The Fundamentals Of Fertility

Fertility is broadly described as the ability to naturally conceive a child in its most basic form. A person's fertility can be affected by a variety of factors, including physiological and environmental impacts.To gain a deeper understanding of fertility and empower your family-building choices, it's crucial to learn about some of the fundamental concepts related to reproductive health and the factors that affect fertility.

1. **Female Fertility:**

The biological functions that determine how the reproductive system conceives and nourishes the developing embryo are referred to as female fertility. Ovulation and menstruation are important aspects in female reproductive health. The ovulation and menstruation cycle lasts approximately 28 days; it is a complex process governed by female hormones that cause a variety of responses, including:

- Menstruation – the shedding of the uterine lining
- The Follicular Phase – the preparation of an ovarian follicle that will mature into an egg
- Ovulation – the development and release of an egg from the ovaries
- The thickening of the uterine lining in advance of pregnancy is known as the "luteal phase."
- Age & Female Fertility:

Although fertility in both men and women is affected by aging, age negatively impacts female fertility significantly more. Fertility in women often peaks in their 20s and early 30s, declining sharply after age 35, which makes conception more challenging.

- Egg Quality:

A person's "ovarian reserve," or the quantity and quality of their eggs, directly affects their ability to conceive. The best chance of forming an embryo, implanting in the uterus, and resulting in a healthy, successful pregnancy is with healthy, high-quality eggs. Because an individual's quantity and quality of eggs decline with age, age is a major contributing factor to inadequate ovarian reserve.Other factors that can influence ovarian reserve include conditions such as:

- Endometriosis – a condition in which the tissue that lines the uterus grows in other places in the pelvic cavity, including the ovaries and fallopian tubes

- PCOS is a hormonal condition that interferes with insulin production and ovulation. Opposition
- Damaged or blocked fallopian tubesOvarian cysts
- Ovarian cyst
- Certain immune disorders
- Obesity
- Cancer treatment (e.g., chemotherapy)
- Heavy alcohol or drug use
- Smoking

2. Male Fertility:

The quality and quantity of sperm in a sample of semen is the main factor used to calculate male fertility. The ability to impregnate can be impacted by having insufficient sperm, sperm with irregular shapes, sperm with poor swimming abilities, or sperm with fragmented DNA.

- Low Sperm Count (Oligospermia):

Oligospermia is the condition in which there is less sperm than normal in the semen (less than 15 million sperm in 1 milliliter of semen), which leaves less sperm available to fertilize the egg.

- Poor Sperm Motility:

The capacity of the sperm to move toward the egg for fertilization is known as sperm motility. Obstacles to sperm motility could make fertilization challenging. The following variables may have a detrimental effect on sperm motility function:

1. Usage of illegal drugs (such as cocaine and cannabis)
2. High environment temperature (heat stress damages sperm)
3. Medical conditions (e.g., varicocele, swelling of the veins in the testicles)

- Abnormal Sperm Morphology:

The term "morphology" describes the shape of the sperm; a distorted sperm may have trouble piercing the egg, which could lead to infertility. The following conditions are known to result in aberrant sperm morphology:

- Certain genetic abnormalities
- Exposure to toxic chemicals
- An increase in testicular temperature
- Infection

3. **Lifestyle and Fertility**

Healthy lifestyle choices can positively impact male and female fertility. Maintaining a healthy body weight, a healthy diet, regular exercise, stress management, managing any underlying conditions (including STIs), and avoiding tobacco, drugs, alcohol, and other toxins can contribute to better male and female reproductive health.

4. **The Window of Fertility:**

Fertility is not a constant; it ebbs and flows. The window of fertility, typically centered around ovulation, the prime opportunity for conception. Recognizing and utilizing this window is foundational for couples on the path to parenthood.

5. **Fertility Testing:**

Fertility testing can provide valuable insights into reproductive health. Tests such as hormone level assessments, semen analysis, and imaging studies can help identify potential challenges and guide fertility interventions.

6. **Medical Interventions:**

In cases where natural conception faces challenges, medical interventions such as fertility medications, assisted reproductive technologies (ART), and in vitro fertilization (IVF) offer viable options. Seeking guidance from fertility specialists becomes crucial at this juncture. When it comes to scheduling an appointment with a fertility specialist,the general rule of thumb is to seek help after a year of trying to conceive if you're under the age of 35. If you're 35 or older, it's generally recommended to see a fertility specialist after six months of trying to conceive. But since each person is unique, there may be circumstances in which you should seek assistance sooner, such as if you are over 40 or have a known reproductive issue.

7. **Emotional Well-being:**

Acknowledging and addressing the emotional aspects of the fertility journey is foundational. The process can be emotionally taxing, and seeking support, whether through counseling, support groups, or open communication with a partner, is integral to navigating the emotional landscape.

The role of nutrition in fertility

In the beautiful tapestry of life, the role of nutrition in fertility is akin to a nurturing embrace, gently guiding the intricate dance toward parenthood. It's not just about what we eat; a significant association winds through the actual texture of our prosperity, impacting the striking excursion of origination and the formation of life.

Nurturing the Foundation:

Think of nutrition as the loving foundation that supports the dream of parenthood. Essential vitamins and minerals become the tender architects, shaping the landscape for the conception and development of healthy eggs and sperm. Supplements like folic corrosive, zinc, and omega-3 unsaturated fats paint the material, adding to the show-stopper of life.

Harmony in Hormones:

In the poetic ballet of fertility, hormonal balance is the music that sets the rhythm of the journey. Nutrition plays the role of a gentle conductor, ensuring the orchestra of hormones harmonizes seamlessly. By providing the body with the right nutrients, we compose the symphony that orchestrates ovulation, sperm production, and the delicate dance of implantation.

Guardians Against Oxidative Stress:

Enter the guardians – antioxidants. Picture them as the valiant protectors shielding eggs and sperm from the tumult of oxidative stress. Fruits, vegetables, and whole grains, adorned in vibrant hues, stand as warriors in this cosmic battle, creating a sanctuary where fertility can bloom.

Weight and Metabolism as Dance Partners:

In the waltz of fertility, weight and metabolism sway gracefully. Too much or too little disrupts the dance. A balanced diet and a dance with physical activity become the partners that guide us, ensuring the rhythm remains steady, supporting the delicate interplay of hormones and menstrual cycles.

Quelling the Inflammatory Symphony:

Life's symphony is susceptible to discordant notes of inflammation. Enter the healers – anti-inflammatory foods. Picture them as the peacemakers, soothing the rhythms within, creating an atmosphere where fertility can find its melody.

A Holistic Embrace:

Yet, nutrition is not a strict conductor; it's a warm embrace. Beyond the scientific ballet, it nurtures our essence. It whispers words of comfort, eases our stresses, and paints smiles on our faces. A well-balanced diet becomes the companion, not just in the journey to conception, but in the blooming of our overall well-being.

In this grand story of fertility, nutrition is the protagonist, the friend who walks beside us. It's a human connection, an ally on the path to parenthood, a reminder that every bite carries the potential to shape a story—our story—of creating life

Lifestyle Factors Affecting Fertility

For the estimated 10-18% of couples affected by infertility, finding the root cause of the problem can be a difficult and lengthy process. This is due to the fact that, generally speaking, female variables or a combination of both are just as likely to be the cause of fertility issues as male causes.

In many cases, infertility is the result of lifestyle factors that compromise reproductive health and make pregnancy far less likely.

Thankfully, the majority of these variables are under your control, which means that you can change or reverse them with just better decisions and improved daily routines. Find out more about the impact of your lifestyle on your ability to conceive as well as your options.

Body weight

One in ten women of reproductive age, or more than six million women in the US, have trouble getting pregnant or maintaining a pregnancy. Being overweight, obese, or noticeably underweight is a direct cause of infertility for a large number of these women.

Being overweight or underweight can make it more difficult to become pregnant because both conditions influence your estrogen levels and disrupt normal ovulation, which is the monthly release of an egg from one of your ovaries.

Normal estrogen levels are necessary for regular ovulation, however being overweight can increase the amount of circulating estrogen, which prevents ovulation in a manner similar to birth control. On the other hand, being underweight may interfere with your body's ability to produce enough estrogen to promote monthly ovulation.

For women on both ends of the spectrum, taking steps toward a healthier weight is often enough to restore normal ovulation and make pregnancy possible.

Nutrition

Although there has been little research on how a woman's nutritional status influences her chances of conceiving, there is plenty of evidence to suggest that eating a balanced diet promotes good body function. functioning and general well-being.

Still, there is no precise "fertility diet" to follow when attempting to conceive. Instead, keep in mind that your body functions best when it is properly fuelled, and your reproductive system is no exception.

That means choosing whole foods like vegetables, fruits, whole grains, proteins, and healthy fats, while limiting or eliminating refined grain products and foods that are rich in added sugars, preservatives, or unhealthy fats.

It's crucial to remember, though, that female fertility has been demonstrated to be hampered by untreated celiac illness (gluten intolerance).

Physical activity

When exercise is necessary to keep your body strong and healthy, it's best to avoid doing too much of it when you're trying to conceive. This is due to the fact that intense exercise may disrupt regular ovulation and lower progesterone levels, which are vital reproductive hormones for conception.

In fact, researchers have found a strong correlation between increased frequency, intensity, and duration of exercise and decreased fertility in women.

Stick to moderate exercise when attempting to conceive, regardless of whether you've always been an athlete or are trying to reduce weight. Women who want to maintain more intense training programs are generally advised to limit vigorous exercise to no more than five hours each week.

Smoking

This gives you even more motivation to give up smoking if you've been having trouble becoming pregnant.

Tobacco use has a number of detrimental effects on female fertility. It can prematurely age your ovaries, deplete your eggs, damage your cervix and fallopian tubes, and increase your risk of having an ectopic pregnancy or miscarriage.

If all of that weren't enough, smoking is also incredibly harmful to a growing fetus and your overall health. Giving up the habit permanently will help you avoid infertility issues, safeguard your pregnancy, and have a healthy child.

Alcohol consumption

It has long been recognized by medical professionals that consuming alcohol in any quantity while pregnant poses a risk to the developing foetus. More recently, it has also been found that alcohol use can drastically lower a woman's fertility.

While the precise mechanism by which alcohol impairs conception is yet unknown, evidence points to possible various interferences of alcohol with proper ovulation.

Because no one knows how much or how little alcohol it takes to interfere with reproductive function, women who are trying to conceive are generally encouraged to avoid alcohol completely.

Other factors

There are other lifestyle variables like being overweight, eating poorly, exercising excessively, smoking, and consuming alcohol that might affect your ability to conceive.

You may have a harder time getting pregnant if you have anxiety, suffer from depression, or live with some other form of chronic psychological stress. If you feel stressed out more often than not, finding ways to relax or seeking support can make a significant difference.

Exposure to harmful substances on a frequent basis can potentially affect fertility. For example, lead in drinking water can affect hormone levels and decrease fertility, and many pesticide chemicals can interfere with normal hormonal function. with reproductive health.

Fertility experts even recommend limiting the amount of caffeine you consume when trying to conceive, although research hasn't yet shown a clear link between too much caffeine and infertility. Just as with alcohol, however, it's better to be safe than sorry when you're doing everything you can to get pregnant.

CHAPTER 2: BUILDING A FERTILITY-FRIENDLY DIET

Choosing the right foods is only the first step in creating a fertility-friendly diet; It transforms into a deliberate and empowering journey in the direction of creating the ideal environment for conception. At its center, this try includes key decisions that go past fulfilling hunger, meaning to feed the complex cycles of conceptive wellbeing.

A menu that has been carefully selected to meet key nutritional requirements is known as a fertility-friendly diet. It is intended to improve fertility. It spins around the thought that food isn't just food yet has a strong effect on hormonal equilibrium, cell wellbeing, and the general prosperity of the two accomplices. This purposeful methodology perceives the significant association among nourishment and the complex dance prompting life as a parent.

Nutrient-dense foods that supply a variety of vitamins, minerals, and antioxidants are the foundation of a fertility-friendly diet. Products of the soil, entire grains, lean proteins, and sound fats structure the foundation, working synergistically to establish a climate helpful for conceptive achievement. Folic acid from leafy greens and legumes supports the early stages of fetal development, while omega-3 fatty acids from sources like fatty fish contribute to hormonal harmony.

Importantly, a diet that is good for fertility promotes mindfulness and moderation. One way to maintain fertility is to avoid reused reflections, sweet and ameliorated carbs. maintaining a healthy weight is essential

In essence, putting together a diet that is good for fertility is a deliberate process that combines nutrients, flavors, and intention. It is an interest in regenerative wellbeing, adjusting dietary decisions to the desire to make a ripe ground where the wonder of origination can unfurl normally and agreeably.

Guidelines for a balanced and fertility-enhancing diet

Exploring the domain of ripeness upgrading sustenance includes an insightful mix of equilibrium, assortment, and deliberate decisions. Here are far reaching rules to direct the formation of an eating regimen that supports generally prosperity as well as ideally upholds the mind boggling cycles of proliferation:

1. Supplement Rich Establishment:

The foundation of a ripeness accommodating eating routine lies in its supplement thickness. Focus on various entire, supplement rich food varieties like natural products, vegetables, entire grains, lean proteins, and dairy or dairy options. These food sources give fundamental nutrients, minerals, and cell reinforcements significant for conceptive wellbeing.

2. Embrace Solid Fats:

Consolidate wellsprings of solid fats, like avocados, nuts, seeds, and olive oil. Omega-3 unsaturated fats, found in greasy fish like salmon, assume a critical part in advancing hormonal equilibrium and supporting general conceptual wellbeing.

3. Ideal Protein Admission:

Guarantee a sufficient admission of great proteins, including lean meats, poultry, fish, eggs, and plant-based sources like vegetables and tofu. Protein is fundamental for cell fix, chemical creation, and the general working of contraceptive organs.

4. Folic Corrosive Concentration:

Folic corrosive, a B-nutrient, is vital for forestalling brain tube imperfections and supporting early fetal turn of events. Mixed greens, vegetables, invigorated grains, and citrus organic products are amazing sources. Its consideration is critical for the two accomplices in bias consideration.

5. Pick Complex Sugars:

Select complex carbs like entire grains, earthy colored rice, and quinoa. These give supported energy, manage glucose levels, and add to hormonal equilibrium, which are all helpful for ripeness.

6. Hydration Matters:

Remaining all around hydrated is fundamental for generally speaking wellbeing, including conceptual wellbeing. Water upholds cell capability, supports supplement transport, and keeps up with hormonal equilibrium.

7. Careful Balance:

While making a fruitfulness accommodating eating routine, balance is critical. Take a stab at a reasonable admission of supplements, staying away from extreme utilization of handled food varieties, sugars, and refined starches. This keeps a sound weight, which is a pivotal calculation fruitfulness.

8. Limit Caffeine and Liquor:

Balance reaches out to caffeine and liquor utilization. Restricting caffeine admission and staying away from exorbitant liquor utilization is prudent, as these substances might possibly affect hormonal equilibrium and richness.

9. Individualized Approach:

Perceive the uniqueness of individual wholesome requirements. Talking with a medical services proficient or a nutritionist can give customized direction, considering explicit dietary necessities and potential ripeness challenges.

10. Bright Range of Produce:

Embrace the energy of a beautiful exhibit of foods grown from the ground. The different colors connote a range of supplements, including cell reinforcements and phytochemicals, which assume an imperative part in killing free extremists and supporting regenerative wellbeing.

11. Incline Towards Plant-Based Proteins:

Consider consolidating more plant-based protein sources like beans, lentils, and tofu. Plant-based proteins offer a range of supplements while frequently being lower in immersed fats, adding to in general cardiovascular wellbeing — a viewpoint complicatedly connected to richness.

12. Zest it Up with Mitigating Spices:

Inject your culinary collection with mitigating spices and flavors like turmeric, ginger, and cinnamon. These culinary wonders upgrade flavor as well as add to a decent provocative reaction, encouraging a climate helpful for origination.

13. Dairy or Dairy Choices:

Incorporate wellsprings of calcium and vitamin D through dairy or invigorated dairy options. These supplements are essential for bone wellbeing as well as for managing hormonal cycles, including those basic for fruitfulness.

14. Careful Desserts:

Fulfill sweet desires carefully. Decide on normally sweet choices like natural products, or enjoy dull chocolate, which satisfies the sweet tooth as well as gives cell reinforcements advantageous to regenerative wellbeing.

15. Supportable Fish Decisions:

In the case of consolidating fish, pick assortments wealthy in omega-3 unsaturated fats and low in mercury. Salmon, trout, and sardines are amazing decisions. These unsaturated fats add to hormonal equilibrium and back the wellbeing of regenerative cells.

Nutrients Crucial For Fertility

For Ladies:

Acid folic: This B nutrient is fundamental for forestalling brain tube surrenders in children, and it likewise assumes a part in sound egg improvement. At least 400 micrograms of folic acid should be taken by pregnant women every day, ideally before conception.

Iron: Iron is required for healthy egg production and ovulation as well as for oxygen transport in the blood. Ladies who are attempting to imagine ought to mean to get 18 milligrams of iron everyday.

D vitamin: This vitamin is necessary for immune system function and bone health, and it may also affect fertility. Ladies who are attempting to imagine ought to expect to get 600 global units (IUs) of vitamin D everyday.

Omega-3 unsaturated fats: These sound fats are significant for mind wellbeing and advancement, and they may likewise further develop ripeness. Omega-3s can be obtained from fatty fish like salmon, tuna, and mackerel or from supplements for pregnant women.

Antioxidants: Cancer prevention agents assist with shielding cells from harm, and they may likewise further develop richness. Whole grains, fruits, and vegetables can provide antioxidants to pregnant women.

For Men:

Zinc: Zinc is necessary for the motility and production of sperm, as well as for the production of testosterone. The recommended daily intake of zinc for men trying to conceive is 11 milligrams.

Selenium: The health and motility of sperm are dependent on this mineral, which may also shield sperm from damage. Men who are attempting to imagine ought to intend to get 55 micrograms of selenium everyday.

C vitamin: This vitamin is an antioxidant that may help improve the quality of sperm and protect them from damage. Men who are attempting to imagine ought to intend to get 90 milligrams of L-ascorbic acid day to day.

E vitamin: This vitamin is an antioxidant that may help improve the quality of sperm and protect them from damage. The recommended daily intake of vitamin E for men trying to conceive is 15 milligrams.

Vitamin Q10: This coenzyme is significant for sperm creation and motility, and it might likewise further develop sperm quality. Coenzyme Q10 can be taken by men trying to conceive through supplements.

Food groups and their fertility benefits

- **Fruits and Vegetables:**

Abundant in vitamins, minerals, and antioxidants, fruits and vegetables form the backbone of a fertility-friendly diet. Leafy greens provide folate, essential for fetal development, while colorful fruits supply antioxidants that combat oxidative stress, nurturing reproductive cells

- **Protein**

Proteins are a major structural and functional macronutrient of our body. They are also required for the production of eggs and sperm. Choose additional plant sources of this crucial vitamin when attempting to conceive. Beans and lentils are not just rich in proteins that support better ovulation, but also contain fiber and folate that is essential in maintaining a good hormonal balance. Additionally, lentils have high quantities of polyamine spermidine, which is thought to assist in the fertilization of eggs by sperm.

for non-vegetarian protein, choose salmon. Salmon is often regarded as a fertility superfood due to its high concentration of omega-3 fatty acids, which assist maintain the health of your reproductive system and keep you fertile.the best possible condition; its high protein content; and the fact that it is nearly devoid of mercury that is found at high levels in many other fish. When attempting to conceive, salmon is a considerably better alternative than red meat, which, due to its high saturated fat content, may make it more difficult to conceive.

- **Healthy Fats**

Moderate consumption of healthy fats from plants is an essential recommendation of the fertility diet.

Saturated fats found in nuts, olives, and grapeseed oil have been demonstrated to lower inflammation, which is essential for increasing ovulation and fertility in women.

Snacking on nuts such as avocados and almonds has additional advantages. Avocados are loaded with nutrients such as vitamin K and potassium that help your body in a variety of ways, including the absorption of vitamins, the management of blood pressure, and more. They also include monounsaturated fats as well as high quantities of dietary fiber and folic acid, both of which are known to be important in the early stages of a woman's pregnancy. Almonds are rich in zinc, vitamin E and L-arginine, vital to the health of the reproductive system, making them one of the best nut options for boosting fertility.

- **Complex Carbs**

Eat more complex carbohydrates and less highly processed foods to improve fertility. Refined carbohydrates, such as those found in cookies and white bread, are readily absorbed and transformed by the body into blood sugar. To minimize blood sugar rises, the pancreas secretes insulin into the bloodstream, and research suggests that high insulin levels may interfere with ovulation.

Complex carbohydrates, such as fruits, vegetables, legumes, and whole grains, are slowly digested and have a more progressive influence on blood sugar and insulin levels. Minimally processed grains are high in fertility-boosting nutrients including vitamin E and B vitamins. The gut microbiota is fed by insoluble fiber, which is plentiful in whole grains, nuts, and vegetables. A healthy gut flora population is important for a healthy metabolism and fertility.

During mid-meal hunger, roasted sunflower seeds can be ingested. They are high in vitamin E and high in important elements including folate and selenium, both of which promote fertility. Additionally, they are an excellent source of omega-6 fatty acids.

- **Whole-Fat Dairy**

Consuming a proper quantity of calcium is critical while attempting to conceive, but not all kinds of calcium are created equal.. The calcium that is included in skim milk and other types of milk with a lower amount of fat does not absorb as well as the calcium that is present in whole-fat dairy products. Additionally, whole milk is a rich source of both protein and vitamin B12. Low-fat dairy has also been found to increase the risk of ovulatory infertility in women. When purchasing dairy products, be certain that the cows are not given hormones or antibiotics.

CHAPTER 3:

BREAKFAST RECIPES

Scrambled eggs and whole grain toast with smoked salmon

- Prep time: 30 minutes
- Cook time:10 minutes
- Serving: 1

INGREDIENTS

- 1 tbsp butter, plus extra for spreading
- 2 large free-range eggs
- 1 tbsp milk
- 1 slice whole meal, bread, toasted
- 2 slices smoked salmon
- salt and freshly ground black pepper

DIRECTIONS

1. Melt the butter in a pot over low heat for the scrambled eggs.

2. Stir in the eggs continuously. Cook the scrambled eggs carefully, no less than 5 minutes, to keep them creamy.

3. Add the milk once the mixture thickens. After removing from the fire, add salt and pepper for seasoning.

4. Place the slice of toast in the center of the platter to serve. Spoon over the scrambled eggs, place the smoked salmon on top and season with lots of black pepper.

NUTRITIONAL INFORMATION

605 kcal, 33 g protein, 17 g carb (including 2 g sugars), 44 g fat (including 21 g saturates), 2 g fiber, and 3 g sodium are included in each meal.

Black beans and avocado on whole-grain toast

- Prep time: 5 minutes
- Serving : 2
- Total time: 5 minutes

INGREDIENTS

- 1 cup canned black beans, no salt added
- ½ avocado
- 2 tbsp water
- 1 tsp chili pepper flakes
- 2 slice whole grain bread

DIRECTIONS

1. Toast your bread of choice.
2. In a blender, combine avocado and rinsed canned black beans.

3. Begin mixing and gradually add 1 tablespoon of water at a time to obtain a smooth, spreadable, creamy consistency.

4. Spread the black bean avocado mixture on two slices of bread and top with a sprinkling of chile peppers to serve.

NUTRITIONAL INFORMATION

Calories: 233 kcal, Carbohydrates: 31g, Protein: 10g, Fat: 9g, Saturated Fat: 1g, Fiber:11g
Sugar:2g

shakshuka

- Prep time: 10 mins
- Cook time: 20 mins
- Total: 30
- Serving: 6 servings

INGREDIENT

- 2 tablespoon of olive oil
- 1 medium onion, diced
- 1 red bell pepper, seeded and diced
- 4 garlic cloves, finely chopped
- 2 teaspoon of paprika
- 1 teaspoon of cumin
- ¼ teaspoon of chili powder
- 128- ounce can whole peeled tomato
- 6 large eggs
- Salt and pepper to taste
- 1 small bunch of fresh cilantro, chopped
- 1 small bunch of fresh parsley, chopped

DIRECTION

1. Heat the olive oil in a large sauté pan over medium heat.Cook for 5 minutes, or until the onion becomes translucent, with the diced bell pepper and onion.

2. Add the spices and garlic, then stir and simmer for an additional minute.

3. Pour in the can of tomatoes and liquid and break down the tomatoes with a big spoon. After adding salt and pepper to taste, bring the sauce to a boil.

4. Make tiny wells in the sauce with your big spoon and crack the eggs into each one. Cook, covered, for 5-8 minutes, or until the eggs are done to your taste.

5. Garnish with chopped cilantro and parsley.

NUTRITION INFORMATION

CALORIES: 146 KCAL | CARBOHYDRATES: 10G | PROTEIN: 7G | FAT: 9G | SATURATED FAT: 2G | FIBER: 2G | SUGAR: 5G

Spiced Chia Porridge with Blueberry Compote

- Prep Time : 5mins
- Cook Time: 10mins
- Total Time: 15mins
- Servings : 2

INGREDIENTS

- 1 cup rolled oats
- 1/2 tsp ground cinnamon
- 1/4 tsp ground cardamom
- 50 g vanilla protein powder optional
- Two cups plant-based milk of choice or soy milk
- 1 tsp vanilla extract
- 1 tbsp maple syrup or sweetener of choice

- 1 tsp chia seeds

Blueberry Chia Compote

- 1.5 cup frozen blueberries
- 1 tbsp water
- 1 tbsp chia seeds

To serve

- 250 g punnet of fresh strawberries, cut in quarters, with the crowns removed
- 1/2 cup coconut yogurt or plant-based yogurt of choice
- maple syrup

DIRECTION

Blueberry Chia Compote

1. Pour water and blueberries into a medium-sized microwave-safe bowl. After three minutes of high heat, stir

2. Heat the mixture for a further minute at a time until it is piping hot and the blueberries have begun to soften.

3. Toss in the chia seeds and mix thoroughly.. Leave to sit for 5-10 minutes until the mixture has thickened.

Spiced Chia Porridge

1. In a small saucepan, add oats, chia, spices, and protein powder (optional). Heat the milk, vanilla essence, and maple syrup in a saucepan over medium heat until the porridge begins to boil.

2. Reduce the heat to low and continue to cook for 5 minutes. If necessary, add more milk to maintain the consistency smooth.

3. Serve the porridge into bowls, top with blueberry compote, fresh strawberries, yogurt and extra maple syrup if desired.

NUTRITIONAL INFORMATION

Calories: 567 kcal | Carbohydrates: 82g | Protein: 35g | Fat: 12g | Saturated Fat: 2g

Avocado toast with Eggs

- Prep time: 5 mins
- Cook time: 5 mins
- Total time: 10 mins
- Serving: 1

INGREDIENTS

- 1 piece multigrain bread or your preferred bread
- ½ whole Avocados mashed
- Lemon juice to taste, in avocado
- Salt and Pepper to taste
- Red Pepper Flakes to taste

Fried Egg

- 1 whole egg
- 2 tsps. butter

Poached Egg

- 1 whole egg

- 1 tsp. vinegar to add in the water when you cook it

Scrambled Egg

- 1 whole egg

- 2 tsps. butter

DIRECTION

1. Use the oven or toaster to toast your bread.

2. Remove the seed from the avocados.

3. Scoop the avocados into a bowl and season with lemon juice, salt, and red pepper flakes.

4. Smash your avocado with a fork to the desired texture. Either leave it lumpy or mash it until it's smooth.

5. Spread it onto your toasted bread.

6. Top with cooked eggs

7. Garnish and enjoy.

NUTRITIONAL INFORMATION:

Calories: 142 kcal | Carbohydrates: 12g | Protein: 4g | Fat: 9g | Saturated Fat: 5g |Fiber: 2g | Sugar: 2g

Scrambled eggs with spinach and Feta

- Prep time: 5 mins
- Cook time: 5 mins
- Total: 10 mins
- Serving : 2

INGREDIENTS

- 4 oz. fresh spinach
- 4 large eggs
- 1 Tbsp butter
- 1 oz. feta
- 1 pinch crushed red pepper
- 1 pinch freshly cracked black pepper
- 1 pinch salt

DIRECTION

1. In a large bowl, crack the eggs, add a pinch of salt, and whisk (I prefer ribbons of white and yellow, but you can whisk until even if preferred)

2. In a large saucepan, melt the butter on medium heat.. Add the chopped spinach and cook until it softens (2-3 minutes). Place the sautéed spinach around the sides of the skillet and pour the eggs in the middle.

3. Roughly slice the spinach into smaller (1-inch) pieces. This step is optional and can be skipped to speed up breakfast. .

4. Gently fold the eggs as the bottom layer solidifies, until the eggs are about 75% solid

5. . Fold the eggs into the sautéed spinach and remove from the heat.The residual heat in the pan will finish cooking the eggs without overcooking or drying them out.

6. Top the eggs with the crumbled feta, a little freshly cracked pepper, and a pinch of crushed red pepper, then serve.

NUTRITIONAL INFORMATION

Calories: 250.75kcal   Carbohydrates: 3.6g
Protein: 16.2g   Fat: 19g   Fiber: 1.3g

Burrito with egg beans and cheese

- Prep time: 10 mins
- Cook time: 5 mins
- Total: 15 mins
- Serving: 4

INGREDIENT

- 8 eggs
- ¼ tsp of each salt and pepper
- 2 tsp of butter
- 1 cup washed and depleted canned dark beans
- 2 tsp of lime juice
- 4 cups of large whole grain flour tortillas, warmed
- ½ cup of prepared tomato salsa
- 2 tsp of chopped fresh cilantro
- ½ cup of shredded cheddar cheese

DIRECTION

1. Whisk eggs with salt and pepper.

2. Melt butter in a large nonstick pan over medium-low heat; add egg mixture. Cook, stirring constantly, for 3 to 5 minutes, or until the egg mixture begins to form soft curds.

3. Mash beans with a potato masher and lime juice.

4. Place tortillas on a clean work area and sprinkle mashed beans down the center of each.

5. Distribute the salsa, scrambled eggs, cilantro, and cheese equally.

6. Fold tortilla bottoms over contents, then fold in edges and roll securely.

7. If preferred, top each tortilla with 1 tbsp (15 mL) guacamole or avocado slices.

NUTRITIONAL INFORMATION:

Calories 470 Kcal, Cab 40g, protein 24g, fats 24g, saturated fat 10g, sugar 2g, fiber 7g

Greek Yogurt with Berries, Nuts and Honey

- Prep time: 5 mins
- Cook time: 0 mins
- Total: 5 mins
- Serving:1

INGREDIENTS

- 6 oz nonfat plain Greek yogurt
- 1 tbsp honey, local preferred
- 1/2 cup fresh berries
- 1 tbsp chopped walnut

DIRECTION

1. In a serving plate, layer yogurt with berries, nuts, and honey.
2. Granola would taste great too

NUTRITIONAL INFORMATION

Serving: 1 bowl, Calories: 250 kcal, Carbohydrates: 35.5 g, Protein: 19.5 g, Fat: 4.5 g, Saturated Fat: 0.5 g, Fiber: 2.5 g, Sugar: 31.5 g

Sweet potato hash with eggs

- Prep time:15 mins
- Cook time: 20 mins
- Total: 35 mins
- Serving: 4 servings

INGREDIENTS

- Cut 4 bacon slices into pieces that are 1/2 inch thick.
- 1 small onion, diced
- 1 red bell pepper, diced
- 1 big peeled and chopped sweet potato into 1/2-inch cubes (about 4 cups cubes)
- 2 cups kale leaves, roughly chopped
- 1/4 teaspoon cumin
- 1/4 teaspoon garlic powder
- 1/4 teaspoon paprika
- salt and pepper, to taste
- 4 eggs

- 1 green onion, sliced

DIRECTION

1. Heat a large saute pan on medium heat. Sauté the bacon until brown and crispy. Remove the bacon with a slotted spoon to a paper towel or small dish.

2. Cook for one minute to soften the chopped onion and red bell pepper in the pan.

3. To the pan, add the diced sweet potato and seasonings. . Cook the sweet potato for 10-12 minutes, stirring often. Cover the pan for the last 5 minutes to soften the sweet potato till it is fork tender.

4. Return the bacon to the pan with the kale and stir for another 1-2 minutes, or until the kale has wilted.

5. Use a spatula to create 4 wells in the hash. Cook until the eggs are done to your taste

by cracking one egg into each well. To speed up the cooking time, cover the pan with a lid.

6. Remove the breakfast hash from the heat. Season with salt and pepper and garnish with green onion slices. Serve immediate

NUTRITIONAL INFORMATION CALORIES:222 KCAL| CARBOHYDRATE:15G PROTEIN: 11G | FAT: 13G | SATURATED FAT: 4G | FIBER: 2G | SUGAR: 4G

Whole-wheat tortillas with beans and salsa

- Prep time:10 mins
- Cook time: 35 mins
- Total : 45 mins
- Serving : 4 servings

INGREDIENTS

- 1 tablespoon olive oil, in addition to something else for brushing
- 1 onion, finely sliced
- 2 garlic cloves, crushed or grated
- 1 tsp smoked sweet paprika
- 1 (400g) tin chopped tomatoes
- 2 cans (400g) kidney or black beans, washed and drained
- 1 (300g) jar mild salsa dip

- 4 coarsely chopped jalapeno chili slices from a jar, plus additional slices to serve (optional)
- 6 medium flour tortillas
- 100g cheddar, grated
- 1 avocado, sliced
- 150ml soured cream
- 2 salad onions, trimmed and finely sliced
- 1 small handful coriander sprigs

DIRECTION

1. Preheat the oven to 200C/180C fan/gas 6. In a large skillet, heat the oil over medium heat and cook the onion for 8-10 minutes, turning constantly, until softened.

2. Cook for one to two minutes after adding the paprika and garlic. Add the chopped tomatoes, salsa, beans, and jalapeños and stir. Once well-seasoned, lower the heat

and let the mixture boil for ten minutes, or until it thickens.

3. pread some oil on the tortillas and place four of them, oil-side down, in an ovenproof 23 x 30 cm dish. Line the edges and bottom of the dish to form a tortilla "bowl."

4. Spoon the tomato mix over the tortillas. Tuck in the sides of the two remaining tortillas and lay them over the mixture, greased side up, to cover it loosely. Add cheese on top and bake for 15 minutes, or until the cheese has melted.

5. Serve topped with the avocado, soured cream, salad onions, coriander, extra jalapeños (if you like) and black pepper.

CHAPTER 4 : LUNCH RECIPE

Quinoa salad with chickpeas, vegetables, and a lemon vinaigrette

- Prep time:10 mins
- Cook time: 15 mins
- Total : 25 mins
- Serving: 2 servings

INGREDIENTS

- 1/2 cup (90 g) dry quinoa rinsed
- 1 cup (240 ml) water
- 1/2 tbsp veggie bouillon powder or a mini cube
- 1 (140 g) cucumber chopped
- 1 small (90 g) red onion chopped

- 1 (100 g) chopped pepper
- 2 (150 g) tomatoes chopped
- 1 small (130 g) chopped zucchini
- 3/4 cup canned chickpeas drained and rinsed
- Lemon vinaigrette

DIRECTION

1. Add 1/2 cup rinsed quinoa to a saucepan, cover it with 1 cup of water, and add 1/2 tbsp of bouillon powder (or a mini bouillon cube).

2. Bring to a boil, then lower to a low heat, cover the saucepan with a lid, and let the quinoa simmer for 15 minutes, or until it has absorbed all of the water, then set aside to cool.

3. In the meantime, cut all of the vegetables into similar-sized pieces.

4. Add the cooled quinoa and all chopped veggies and chickpeas to a medium-large bowl

5. .Drizzle with a lemon vinaigrette (or dressing of choice), stir, serve, and enjoy!

NUTRITIONAL INFORMATION

Calories 312 Kcal, Carbohydrates 55g, protein 14g, fat 5g, saturated fat 1g, sugar 9g, fiber 11g

Lentil Soup

- Prep time: 15minute

- Cook time: 30 minutes

- Total: 45 minutes

- Serving: 8 servings

INGREDIENTS

- 2 teaspoon of olive oil

- 1 medium onion, chopped

- 3 cloves garlic, minced

- 2 medium carrots, peeled and chopped

- 2 celery ribs, chopped

- 14- ounce can crushed or diced tomatoes

- 2 cups dry green or brown lentils

- 7 cups vegetable broth

- 1/2 teaspoon ground cumin

- 1/2 teaspoon ground coriander

- 1 teaspoon smoked paprika

- 1 teaspoon salt, or to taste

- 3 cups baby spinach or kale, cut into ribbons

- 1 lemon, juiced (about 2 tablespoons)

DIRECTION

1. Heat the olive oil in a big saucepan over medium heat..

2. Add the onions, garlic, carrots and celery. Cook for about 4-5 minutes, stirring constantly.

3. Now add the canned tomatoes (with juices), lentils, vegetable broth, cumin, coriander, and smoked paprika to the pot.. Stir to incorporate everything.

4. Bring to a boil, then lower heat to a simmer and cook for about 30 minutes, until the lentils are tender and the soup has thickened.

5. Blend a couple times in the saucepan with an immersion blender for a creamier

texture. Alternatively, place 1-2 cups of the soup in a standard blender and puree until smooth before returning to the pot.

6. Stir in the spinach and lemon juice. It will only take a minute for the spinach to wilt. Season with salt to taste.

NUTRITIONAL INFORMATION

Serving: 1 serving | Calories: 236 kcal | Carbohydrates: 38g | Protein: 13g | Fat: 4g | Saturated Fat: 1g Fiber: 16g | Sugar: 7g

Salmon with roasted vegetables

- Prep time:15 mins
- Cook time: 30 mins
- Total: 45mins
- Serving:4 servings

INGREDIENTS

- Peel, cut in half, and chop one red onion into 1-inch pieces.
- Cut two medium zucchini in half lengthwise, then cut into half moon shapes with a knife. Another name for zucchini is courgettes.
- Two delicious red peppers, peeled and sliced into 1-inch segments
- 1 can chickpeas, drained and rinsed that's about 14 ounces or 400 grams but you can use more or less depending on tastes and appetite

- 2 tablespoons mild olive oil

- 1 teaspoon Harissa or to taste check this is gluten free if required

- 4 salmon filets, skinless and boneless if possible. If you want, use a side of salmon and chop it into serving size pieces after it has been cooked.

- chopped flat leaf parsley to garnish

DIRECTION

1. Preheat the oven to 400°F (200°C or 180°C for fan ovens).

2. On a baking sheet/sheet pan, arrange the onion, zucchini, red peppers, and chickpeas.

3. Mix the oil and the Harissa together.

4. Toss the veggies with three-quarters of the oil and spice combination.

5. Place the veggies on a baking sheet in an equal layer and bake for 20 minutes.

6. Remove the skillet from the oven and stir the veggies with a spatula once more.

7. Nestle the salmon filets or side of salmon amongst the vegetables.

8. Brush the remaining oil and spice mixture over the fish.

9. Bake for 10 minutes for salmon filets or 15 to 18 minutes for a side of salmon, until the salmon is cooked through and flakes easily with a fork.

10. Serve garnished with flat leaf parsley.

NUTRITIONAL INFORMATION

Carbs 19g, fats 18g, protein 42g, calories 451Kcal

Stir-fried chicken served with vegetables and brown rice

- Prep time:10 mins
- Cook time: 20 mins
- Total: 30 minutes
- Serving: 6 servings

INGREDIENTS

- 1/3 cup oyster sauce
- 3 tablespoons low-sodium soy sauce, divided, plus more to taste (substitute tamari for gluten-free)
- 2 tbsp each canola oil, grapeseed oil, and peanut oil
- 1 pound boneless, skinless chicken breast cut into bite-sized 1-inch pieces
- 2 tablespoons unsalted butter
- 4 large eggs lightly beaten

- 3 cups chopped fresh veggies of your choosing (I use 8 ounces of mushrooms or 1 red bell pepper with a small head of broccoli)
- 12 ounces frozen peas and carrots thawed
- 3 garlic cloves minced
- 2 1/2 cups COLD cooked brown rice break up large clumps with your fingers
- 2.3 oz of finely chopped green onions (approximately 4 medium)
- Red pepper flakes or Sriracha, or hot sauce of choice (optional)

DIRECTION

1. In a small mixing bowl, combine the oyster sauce and 2 tablespoons soy sauce

2. Place aside. Keep a large basin or plate near the burner, as well as a large, flexible rubber spatula.

3. Heat a 12-inch nonstick skillet over medium heat for about 2 minutes, or until hot

4. . Add 1/2 tablespoon butter and swirl to coat the bottom of the pan. Add the eggs. Cook without stirring for approximately 20 seconds, or until they just begin to set. Scramble and break the eggs into bite-sized pieces using a spatula.

5. Continue to cook, stirring constantly now, until eggs are just cooked through but not yet browned, about 1 additional minute. Place the eggs in a basin and set aside. With a paper towel, clean the skillet.

6. Return the skillet to the heat and bring it up to high. Warm the skillet for about 1 minute, or until it is good and hot. Swirl in 1 tablespoon of canola oil to coat.

7. Combine the chicken and the remaining 1 tablespoon soy sauce in a mixing bowl.

Cook, tossing periodically, for 4 minutes, or until the chicken is thoroughly cooked through. Combine with the eggs in a mixing basin.

8. Add the remaining 1 tablespoon oil to the skillet.Cook until the fresh veggies are crisp-tender, about 4 to 5 minutes.

9. 1 1/2 teaspoons remaining butter, peas, and carrots. Cook, stirring constantly, for 30 seconds.

10. Cook until the garlic is aromatic, about 30 seconds (do not let the garlic burn!).

11. Mix in the brown rice and oyster sauce. Cook, stirring regularly and breaking up any leftover rice clumps, until the mixture is well cooked, about 2 minutes.

12. Combine the reserved eggs/chicken with the green onions. Cook and stir for 1 minute more, or until the mixture is thoroughly cooked through

13. Serve immediately with a sprinkle of red pepper flakes, a splash of spicy sauce, and more soy sauce to taste.

NUTRITIONAL INFORMATION

SERVING:1(of6)CALORIES:368kcal, CARBOHYDRATES:33g PROTEIN: 26gFAT: 15gSATURATED FAT: 4g

Tofu Scramble

- Cook time: 10 mins

- Total: 10 mins

- Serving: 2 servings

INGREDIENTS

- 1 tablespoon olive oil

- (1) 16-ounce block firm tofu

- 2 tablespoons nutritional

- 1/2 teaspoon salt, or more to taste

- 1/4 teaspoon turmeric

- 1/4 teaspoon garlic powder

- 2 tablespoons non-dairy milk, unsweetened and unflavored

DIRECTION

1. In a medium saucepan, heat the olive oil. Mash the tofu block in the pan with a potato masher or a fork. You may also use your hands to crumble it into the pan.

2. Cook, stirring regularly, for 3-4 minutes, or until the tofu's water has almost evaporated.

3. Now, combine the nutritional yeast, salt, turmeric, and garlic powder in a mixing bowl. Cook for 5 minutes, stirring regularly.

4. Pour in the nondairy milk and whisk to combine. Serve immediately with sliced avocado, spicy sauce, parsley, steaming greens, bread, or other breakfast item of choice.

NUTRITIONAL INFORMATION

Serving: 1 serving | Calories: 288 kcal | Carbohydrates: 9g | Protein: 24g | Fat: 18g | Saturated Fat: 2g | Fiber: 4g | Sugar: 1g

Creamy tomato soup with grilled cheese sandwiches

- Prep time: 20 mins
- Cook time: 1 hour
- Total : 1 hour 20 mins
- Serving: 8 Servings

INGREDIENTS

- 12 kilogram (3 pound) tomatoes Use ripe, seasonal tomatoes or entire canned tomatoes instead. San Marzano tomatoes are the best, but any decent quality Italian tomato will do.
- 2 tbsp balsamic vinegar
- 2 tbsp olive oil
- 1 tbsp sugar
- 1 tsp salt
- 2 red onions finely chopped

- 2 garlic cloves finely chopped

- ½ cup fresh basil

- 2 tsp tomato paste

- 8 cups vegetable / chicken stock

- ½ cup cream

- salt & black pepper to taste

- fresh basil to serve for the grilled cheese sandwich

- 2 slices bread per person

- 2 cups grated mozzarella

- 2 cups grated mature

- cheddar butter

DIRECTION

1. Preheat the oven to 200°C/390°F.

2. In a roasting pan, combine the tomatoes (and any liquids if using canned tomatoes) with the Balsamic vinegar, olive oil, sugar, and salt. Stir to combine and place in the oven for

25-30 minutes until the tomatoes are broken down and have started to caramelize.

3. Sauté the onions in olive oil in a large saucepan until transparent and aromatic. Fry for another minute after adding the garlic and basil.

4. Add the roasted tomatoes, tomato paste and sugar. Pour in the stock and stir to mix all of the ingredients.

5. Lower the heat and cover the pot. Allow to simmer for 10 minutes.

6. Remove the soup from the heat and stir it together.

7. Add the cream and season to taste.

8. To prepare the grilled cheese sandwiches, combine the mozzarella and cheddar cheeses. Add 12 cup cheese to half of the bread slices.. Sandwich with the remaining bread. Butter both sides generously

9. Cook until the cheese is melted and the sandwiches are golden brown on both sides in a nonstick pan over medium heat.

10. With the grilled cheese sandwiches, serve the tomato soup with a swirl of cream and fresh basil leaves.

NUTRITIONAL INFORMATION

Calories: 479 kcal | Carbohydrates: 41g | Protein: 22g | Fat: 26g | Saturated Fat: 13g |Fiber: 5g | Sugar: 12g

Salmon with quinoa and roasted vegetables

- Cook time:25 min
- Additional time: 25 mins
- Total: 50 mins
- Serving:4 servings

INGREDIENTS

- A delicata squash, either little or big (approximately 1 pound), should be split, seeded, and cut into 1-inch slices.
- 4 cups cauliflower florets
- 6 small shallots, quartered
- 3 tablespoons extra-virgin olive oil, divided
- ¾ teaspoon salt, divided
- ½ teaspoon ground pepper, divided
- 1 ¼ cups water

- ¾ cup red or white quinoa
- One pound of wild Alaskan salmon filet, divided into four halves after skinning
- Olive oil or canola oil cooking spray
- 3 tablespoons lemon juice
- 2 tablespoons maple syrup
- ¼ cup chopped walnuts, toasted

DIRECTIONS

1. Preheat the oven to 425 degrees F.
2. On a wide rimmed baking sheet, toss the squash, cauliflower, and shallots with 2 tablespoons oil and 1/4 teaspoon each of salt and pepper
3. Roast the veggies for 20 to 25 minutes, tossing once or twice, or until they are soft and browned in places.
4. In the meanwhile, add water to a small saucepan and bring it to a boil. Re-boil the

quinoa after adding it. Simmer on low, covered, for 12 to 15 minutes, or until the water is absorbed. Take off the heat source.

5. Once the veggies are soft, shift them to one side of the pan and put the salmon in the space that is left.

6. Coat the salmon with a thin layer of cooking spray and season with 1/4 teaspoon each salt and pepper. Roast for 4 to 6 minutes, or until the salmon is opaque throughout.

7. In a separate dish, mix together the remaining 1 tablespoon oil, lemon juice, maple syrup, and 1/4 teaspoon salt. Present the quinoa, salmon, and veggies with a dressing drizzle and walnuts on top.

NUTRITIONAL INFORMATION

Calories 499 Kcal, carbs 47g, Fats 22g, protein 32g, Dietary Fiber 9g, Added Sugars 7g,Total Sugars 14g,

Chicken salad with grapes, celery, and walnuts

- Prep time: 15 mins
- Total time: 15 mins
- Serving: 6 servings

INGREDIENTS

- 2 cups of cooked chicken shredded (such as rotisserie)
- 1/3 cup Greek yogurt, sour cream, or mayonnaise;
- 2 tablespoons fresh parsley chopped
- 1/4 cup red onion finely diced
- 1/2 cup red grapes quartered or halved, depending on size
- 1/2 cup celery diced
- 1/4 cup walnuts chopped

- One-half tsp kosher salt, plus extra if necessary
- 1/4 tsp black pepper, plus extra, if necessary

DIRECTION

1. Combine the 2/3 cup of mayonnaise, 1/2 teaspoon of salt, 1/2 teaspoon of black pepper, and 2 tablespoons of freshly chopped parsley in a large bowl.
2. Add the shredded chicken (2 cups), halved or quartered grapes (1/2 cup), diced celery (1/2 cup), chopped walnuts (1/4 cup), and diced red onion (1/4 cup). Stir well to combine
3. Serve over a green salad, over lettuce wraps, or on sandwiches with toasted bread.

NUTRITIONAL INFORMATION

Calories: 292kcal | Carbohydrates: 4g | Protein: 13g | Fat: 25g | Saturated Fat: 4g |Fiber: 1g | Sugar: 3g

Vegetable stir-fry with tofu and brown rice

- Prep time:20 mins:
- Cook time: 15 mins
- Total time: 35 mins
- Serving: 4 servings

INGREDIENTS

- 2 tablespoons olive oil
- 3 cloves garlic, minced
- 1 piece fresh ginger, peeled and coarsely chopped (3 inches)
- 1 medium red bell pepper, peeled and sliced into 1-inch slices
- 1 medium yellow bell pepper, peeled and sliced into 1-inch slices
- 3 cups cooked brown rice

- 3 tablespoons reduced-sodium soy sauce
- 1 teaspoon toasted sesame oil
- Coarse salt and pepper, to taste
- 3 scallions, halved lengthwise and thinly sliced

DIRECTIONS

1. In a large pan or wok, heat the olive oil over medium-high heat.Stir in the garlic and ginger for 30 seconds, or until fragrant.
2. Stir-fry the tofu for 2 minutes, or until golden brown. Cook, stirring constantly, until the red and yellow peppers are crisp-tender, approximately 3 minutes.
3. Cook, stirring periodically, until the rice is well heated, about 3 minutes. Stir in sesame oil. Season with salt and pepper; garnish with scallions. Serve hot.

NUTRITIONAL INFORMATION

Serving Size: 1 serving, Calories: 489, Sodium: 488 mg Fat:17 g, Saturated Fat: 2 g, Carbohydrates: 64 g, Fiber:7g, Protein: 27 g

Black bean burgers on whole-wheat buns

- Prep Time: 5 minutes
- Cook Time: 10 minute
- Total time:15 minutes
- Serving:4 servings

INGREDIENTS

- 1 cup old-fashioned rolled oats
- ½ cup walnut pieces
- 14 inch fresh turmeric piece (or 14 teaspoon ground) grated
- ½ cup red onion chopped
- ⅓ cup mushrooms chopped

- 1 12 cup cooked or 1 15-ounce cleaned and drained BPA-free can or Tetra Pak salt-free black beans
- 2 tablespoons tahini or almond butter
- 1 tablespoon ground flaxseeds
- 1 tablespoon nutritional yeast
- 1 tablespoon fresh parsley chopped
- 2 teaspoons white miso paste
- 1 teaspoon onion powder
- ½ teaspoon garlic powder
- ½ teaspoon smoked paprika
- 1 teaspoon Savory Spice Blend

DIRECTION

1. Preheat the oven to 375°F.
2. In a food processor, pulse the oats, walnuts, and turmeric until finely ground. Pulse in the

onion, mushrooms, beans, tahini, and flaxseeds until fully blended.

3. Add the other ingredients and pulse until fully combined.

4. Pinch a small amount of the mixture between your thumb and index finger to see whether it holds together.

5. Add additional oats if the mixture is too moistAdd a tablespoon of water at a time if the mixture is too dry.Divide the mixture into four equal parts on a work surface.

6. Shape each into a patty about ½-inch thick and transfer to a plate. Refrigerate for 30 minutes.

7. Line a baking sheet with a silicone mat or parchment paper and arrange the burgers on it. Bake for 25 minutes, or until heated and gently browned. Serve hot, as desired

NUTRITIONAL INFORMATION

Serving size: 1 burger patty, Calories: 149 kcal, Fat: 2 g, Saturated fat: 1 g, Carbohydrates: 28 g, Fiber: 8 g,   Sugar: 1   g   Protein: 8   g

CHAPTER 5: DINNER RECIPE

Lentil pasta with marinara sauce and a side salad:

- Prep time: 15 minutes
- Cook time: 45 minutes
- Total time: 1 hour
- Serving: 6 servings

INGREDIENTS

- 1 tablespoon olive oil
- 1 cup (about) finely chopped yellow onion

- 1 carrot, coarsely chopped (about 1/2 cup)
- 1 celery stalk , finely chopped
- 3 garlic cloves , minced
- 1 teaspoon dried basil
- 1 teaspoon dried oregano
- 1/2 teaspoon crushed red pepper flakes (optional; for spice)
- 3/4 cup dry green lentils
- 1 tablespoon maple syrup
- 1 can crushed tomatoes (28 oz) (no salt added)
- 2 1/2 cups water
- fine sea salt

DIRECTIONS

1. Warm the olive oil in a large 6-quart saucepan over medium-high heat. Cook until the onion, carrot, and celery are soft.

2. Stir in the garlic, basil, oregano, and red pepper flakes until combined.

3. Add the lentils, maple syrup, smashed tomatoes, water, and 1 teaspoon of salt to the veggies. (If the tomatoes are unsalted, use half the salt at first to be on the safe side.) Bring the liquid to a boil after thoroughly stirring it.

4. Reduce the heat to a low simmer and cook the sauce, uncovered, for 40 to 45 minutes, or until the lentils are cooked.

5. Stir occasionally to ensure that nothing clings to the bottom of the pot and that the liquid does not evaporate too soon. (If the heat is turned up too much, the liquid may evaporate too quickly.)

6. The lentils are done when they can be readily crushed with a fork on the edge of the saucepan. Season the sauce with additional salt to taste. (I normally add another 1

teaspoon at a time, starting with 1/2 teaspoon.) You may also add a squeeze of fresh lemon or a splash of white wine to brighten the sauce. of balsamic vinegar, if you prefer.

7. Serve warm, with your favorite cooked noodles. The remaining sauce may be refrigerated in an airtight jar for up to a week or frozen for up to 3 months.

NUTRITIONAL INFORMATION

Calories: 123 kcal, Carbohydrates: 19g, Protein: 6g, Fat: 3g, Saturated Fat: 1g, Fiber: 8g, Sugar

Turkey meatballs with spaghetti squash and a side salad

- Prep time:30 mins ,
- cook time: 30 mins
- total: 1 hour,
- serving: 8 servings

INGREDIENT

- 1 pounds spaghetti squash about 2-3
- 1/4 cup water
- 2 tablespoons coconut oil divided (could sub olive oil)
- 1/2 cup fresh parsley divided
- 1 teaspoon italian seasoning
- 1/2 teaspoon onion powder
- 1/2 teaspoon salt

- 1/2 teaspoon pepper

- Optional but tasty: 1 tablespoon coarsely chopped red pepper

- 1 pound dark ground turkey

- 1 28-ounce can crushed tomatoes, no salt

- 2 cloves garlic minced

- 1/4 teaspoon crushed red pepper to taste

DIRECTION

Spaghetti Squash

1. Cut your squash in half lengthwise and scrape out the seeds. Place the squash face down in a roasting pan and cover with water.

2. Roast at 400 degrees F. for about 35-45 minutes, until tender and a knife can be inserted easily through the flesh of squash. Set aside to cool in the pan once finished.

3. Once cool, scoop out spaghetti squash with a fork and place in a big bowl.

Turkey Meatballs

1. Begin prepping the turkey meatballs while the squash is cooking.
2. In a large bowl, add 1/4 cup parsley, 1/2 teaspoon italian seasoning, onion powder, red pepper, 1/2 teaspoon salt, and 1/4 teaspoon pepper.
3. Make 2 tablespoon sized meatballs. You should get about 12 meatballs. Heat the coconut oil in a large skillet and cook the meatballs on medium low until completely cooked and browned, about 20 minutes. Turn off heat and set aside.

Tomato Sauce

1. Cook for around one minute on medium low heat in a medium sized stock pot with one tablespoon extra virgin olive oil and garlic. Combine the crushed tomato sauce, 1/2 teaspoon Italian spice, and salt in a mixing bowl.

2. Allow flavors to simmer and blend for around 10 minutes. Add meatballs to the sauce.

3. Toss some (1-2 tablespoons) ghee or extra virgin olive oil into the spaghetti squash and combine. Enjoy some of the meatballs and sauce combination on top of the spaghetti squash!

NUTRITIONAL INFORMATION

AmountPerServing,   Calories1019   ,Fat107g, SaturatedFat:10g   Carbohydrates   3g   Sugar   1g, Protein 13g

Shrimp scampi with whole-wheat pasta

- Prep time: 10 minutes

- Cook time: 15 minutes

- Total: 25 minutes

- Serving: 4 servings

INGREDIENTS

- Salt

- 12 ounces whole-wheat spaghetti

- ¼ cup olive oil

- 1 pound large shrimp, peeled and deveined

- 4 large cloves garlic, minced

- ½ teaspoon crushed red pepper

- ½ cup dry white wine

- ½ cup finely chopped fresh parsley

DIRECTION

1. Bring a large pot of salted water to boil. Cook until the spaghetti is al dente, about 10 minutes, according to the package guidelines.

2. Warm the oil in a big pan over medium-high heat while the spaghetti cooks. Cook, rotating once, until shrimp are cooked through, about 2 minutes total. Place on a platter.

3. Mix in the garlic, crushed red pepper, wine, and 1/2 teaspoon salt. salt to skillet and simmer 1 minute. Stir in shrimp.

4. Drain pasta, reserving 1/2 cup cooking water. Toss pasta with shrimp mixture and parsley. Add reserved cooking water 1 Tbsp. at a time as needed to moisten. Serve hot

NUTRITIONAL INFORMATION

Per Serving: 591 calories; fat 18g; saturated fat 2g; protein 34g; carbohydrates 67g; fiber 8g; cholesterol 172mg;

Roasted pork chops with apples and sweet potatoes

- Prep time: 10 mins
- cook time: 30 mins
- total: 40 mins
- serving:4 servings

INGREDIENTS

- Spice Rub
- 1 tablespoon coconut sugar (or brown sugar)
- 2 teaspoons paprika
- 1 ½ teaspoons chili powder
- 2 teaspoons fresh thyme (or 1 teaspoon of dried thyme)
- 2 tsp. fresh chopped rosemary (or 1 tsp. dried rosemary)
- 1 ½ teaspoons garlic powder

- ½ teaspoon kosher salt
- ¼ teaspoon pepper
- Pork Chops
- 3 large sweet potatoes peeled and diced small
- 2 tablespoons olive oil
- ½ teaspoon kosher salt
- 1 tablespoon fresh rosemary chopped (or 1 teaspoon dry rosemary)
- 4 pork chops at least 1 inch thick
- 1 large apple (or 2 small apples) diced

DIRECTION

1. Preheat the oven to 425°F and line sheet pan with parchment paper or aluminum foil.
2. Spread the sweet potatoes on a large sheet pan and drizzle with olive oil, salt and pepper. Cook in a preheated oven for 15 minutes.

3. Prepare the pork chops as they cook. Combine the spice rub in a small basin. Rub the ingredients into both sides of the pork chops.

4. When the potatoes are done, arrange them on one side and the pork chops on the other. Toss the apples with the sweet potatoes.

5. To allow for carryover cooking, roast for another 12-15 minutes, or until the sweet potatoes are soft and the pork achieves an internal temperature of slightly about 145°F. Cook time will vary based on the size of the pork chops.

NUTRITIONAL INFORMATION

Serving: 1g | Calories: 478 kcal | Carbohydrates: 33g | Protein: 49.5g | Fat: 16g | Cholesterol: 132.2mg |Fiber: 5.4g | Sugar: 13.2g

Shrimp scampi with zucchini noodles

- Prep time: 15 minutes.

- Cook time: 10 minutes

- total: 25minutes.

- Serving:4serving

  INGREDIENT

- 1 tablespoon unsalted butter

- 1 tablespoon olive oil

- 1 shallot finely chopped

- 4 minced garlic cloves (approximately 1 1/2 teaspoons)

- 1 pound large raw shrimp peeled and deveined with tails on (fresh or frozen and thawed)

- 1 teaspoon kosher salt

- 1/2 teaspoon red pepper flakes

- 1/4 cup white wine or chicken broth (low sodium)

- Zest of 1/2 lemon

- 1/4 cup freshly squeezed lemon juice
- 1 1/2 pounds zucchini noodles from about 4 medium zucchini1/4 cup chopped fresh parsley leaves
- 1/4 cup chopped fresh parsley leaves
- 2 tablespoons freshly grated Parmesa

DIRECTION

1. In a large pan over medium-low heat, melt the butter and olive oil. Cook until the shallot begins to soften, about 3 minutes. Cook for 30 seconds after adding the garlic.

2. Combine the shrimp, salt, red pepper flakes, and black pepper in a mixing bowl. Sauté for 3 minutes, or until the shrimp are starting to cook but remain translucent.

3. Combine the chicken broth, lemon zest, and lemon juice in a mixing bowl. Bring the

shrimp to a boil and simmer for 1 minute, or until they are totally opaque and cooked through

4. Combine the zucchini noodles and parsley in a mixing bowl. Toss the noodles with the shrimp to cover with the garlic-lemon sauce and cook until barely warmed through. . (Do not overcook or the zucchini noodles will become mushy.) Sprinkle with parsley and Parmesan. Serve warm.

NUTRITIONAL INFORMATION

CALORIES:224kcalCARBOHYDRATES:9g PROTEIN: 27gFAT: 9gSATURATED FAT: 3gCHOLESTEROL: 295 mg FIBER: 2gSUGAR: 5g

Chicken baked in the oven with sweet potatoes and Brussels sprouts

- Prep time: 15 minutes
- Cool time: 32 minutes
- Total: 47 minutes
- Serving: 4 servings

INGREDIENTS

- 20 oz. sweet potatoes, peeled and diced into 3/4-inch cubes
- 16 oz. brussels sprouts, bottoms trimmed, halved
- 2 Tbsp olive oil
- Salt and freshly ground black pepper
- 5 slices bacon, diced
- 1 1/2 lbs. chicken breasts, boneless and skinless, chopped into 1 1/4-inch cubes

- 1/2 medium red onion, diced into chunks

- 3 garlic cloves, minced

- 1 Tbsp minced fresh rosemary

- 2 Tbsp minced fresh parsley (optional)

- 3 Tbsp store-bought or homemade** balsamic glaze

DIRECTION

1. Preheat oven to 400 degrees. Apply nonstick cooking spray to an 18 by 13-inch baking sheet that has a rim.

2. Place sweet potatoes and brussels sprouts on baking sheet. Olive oil should be drizzled on and then tossed to coat evenly.

3. After covering everything with bacon, bake for fifteen minutes in a preheated oven. Remove from oven.

4. Toss to cover evenly, then add the chicken, red onions, garlic, and rosemary. Season with salt and pepper. Spread evenly, being careful not to overlap the chicken pieces.

5. Put the chicken back in the oven and continue to roast it for a further 17 to 20 minutes, or until the center of the thickest pieces registers 165.

6. Pour balsamic glaze over everything, or each serving, top with parsley, and serve right away

NUTRITIONAL INFORMATION

Calories   576 Kcal , Fat 22g Saturated Fat : 5g, Carbohydrates   47g,   protein: 40g,   Fiber   9g, sugar:11g

Tuna noodle casserole with whole-wheat bread

- Prep time: 10 mins
- cook time: 1 hour
- total: 1h10 minutes.
- Serving: 1 serving

INGREDIENTS

- Six ounces of egg noodles or no-yolk noodles
- 1 tbsp butter
- 1 medium onion, minced fine
- 3 tbsp flour, or gluten free flour
- 1 3/4 cups fat free chicken broth
- 1 cup 1% milk
- 1 ounce sherry, optional
- 10 ounces sliced baby bella mushroom

- 1 cup frozen petite peas, thawed
- 2 drained 5 ounce cans tuna in water
- 4 ounces Cabot 50% reduced fat sharp cheddar
- 2 tbsp parmesan cheese
- 2 tbsp whole wheat seasoned breadcrumbs
- fresh parsley, chopped for garnish

DIRECTION

1. Cook the noodles in salted water until al dente, or 2 minutes undercooked. Set aside.
2. Melt the butter in a large deep skillet. Cook until the onions are tender, about 5 minutes, over medium heat
3. .Cook for an additional 2-3 minutes on medium-low heat after adding the flour and a touch of salt.

4. Preheat the oven to 375 degrees Fahrenheit. Spray a 9 x 12 casserole dish lightly with butter-flavored cooking spray.

5. Slowly whisk in the chicken broth until thoroughly blended, then raise the heat to medium and whisk for 30 seconds before adding the milk and bringing to a boil.

6. When it begins to boil, add the sherry, mushrooms, and tiny peas, season with salt and pepper to taste, and cook on medium, stirring regularly, until it thickens (approximately 7 to 9 minutes).

7. Add drained tuna, stirring another minute.

8. Remove from the heat and stir in the reduced fat sharp cheddar until it melts. Mix the noodles in the sauce until they are uniformly covered.

9. Pour into the casserole and top with parmesan cheese and breadcrumbs. Top with a little

more cooking spray and bake for about 25 minutes.

10. Broil for a few minutes to crisp up the crumbs (be cautious not to burn).

NUTRITIONAL INFORMATION

Serving: 1 /6th of casserole, Calories: 318kcal, Carbohydrates: 34.3 g, Protein: 27.3g, Fat: 7 g, Saturated Fat: 4 g, Cholesterol:34 mg,Fiber: 3.6 g, Sugar: 6 g

Chicken enchiladas with black beans, corn, and salsa

- Prep time: 15 minutes.
- Cook time: 30 minutes.
- total time: 40 minutes.
- Serving: 4 servings

INGREDIENTS

- 2-3 boneless skinless chicken thighs or breasts from the pantry, cooked and shredded
- 1 cup Wholesome Pantry Organic black beans
- 1 cup corn
- 2 cups Mild Cheddar Wholesome Pantry Organic Fancy Shredded Cheese
- Frontera Red Chili Enchilada Sauce
- Frontera salsa I used their Jalapeño Cilantro

- 12 corn tortillas

DIRECTION

1. Preheat oven to 350 degrees
2. Coat a 13x9 baking dish with nonstick spray and layer with a cup of the salsa.
3. Throw your chicken in a skillet and cook on low.
4. Combine the black beans, corn, 1 cup of cheese, and 1 cup of enchilada sauce in a mixing bowl.
5. Simmer on low until heated through.
6. Warm tortillas in the microwave a few at a time between 2 damn paper towels for 30 seconds.
7. 1/4 cup of the mixture should be spooned onto one side of the tortilla.
8. Place seam side down in a baking tray and roll up.

9. Pour enchilada sauce on top and sprinkle it with the remaining cup of cheese.

10. Bake for 20 minutes, covered with foil..

11. Remove foil and broil and about 5 minutes.

12. Add toppings of choice.Enjoy remaining salsa with chips!

NUTRITIONAL INFORMATION

Per serving: Calories: 641, Total Fat: 34.5g, Sat. 16.5g fat, 118 mg cholesterol, 2,084mg sodium, 51g carbs, 3g fiber, 5g sugar, 31g protein

Curried carrot shorba

- Prep time:10 mins.
- Cook time 30 mins.
- Total time : 40 mins
- serving: 4 servings

INGREDIENTS

- 12 whole Almonds, Soaked Overnight
- 12 whole Cashews, Soaked Overnight
- 2 cups Vegetable Broth (or Water)
- 2 cups Carrots, Peeled And Roughly Chopped
- 1 whole Potato, Roughly Chopped
- 2 teaspoons Ginger, grated
- 3 cloves Garlic, Minced
- 2 teaspoons Finely Chopped Green Chili, Hot
- ½ teaspoons Salt

- ¼ teaspoons Pepper

- 1 teaspoon Paprika Or Chipotle Powder

- 1 teaspoon Extra-Virgin Oil

- 2 teaspoons Butter

- 1 whole Onion, Cut In Half Lengthwise Then Cut Into Thin Slices

- ¼ cups Sour Cream

DIRECTION

1. Drain the almonds and cashews after soaking them in a bowl of water overnight. Set aside.

2. Take a pressure cooker and add the broth or water. Add the carrots, potatoes, almonds, cashews, ginger, garlic, and green chilies now.

3. Set your pressure cooker according to the manufacturer's instructions. Depending on the sort of stovetop pressure cooker you're using,

bring the pressure cooker to high pressure over high heat, then reduce the heat to stabilize the pressure. Keep the time setting for 10 minutes. Turn off the heat and let the cooker cool down.

4. Blend the cooked veggies and nuts into a smooth puree in a food processor.

5. Fill a pot halfway with purée. Season with salt, pepper, and paprika. Bring to a boil before lowering to a low heat for 10 minutes.

6. Meanwhile, in a separate saucepan, add in the olive oil and butter and heat over medium heat until the butter melts. Into the melted butter mixture, add the sliced onions and saute on high flame until the onions are caramelized and golden brown. Take 2 teaspoons of the cooked onion and save aside for garnish.

7. Mix in the remainder of the onions into the soup. Add the sour cream and stir. Remove

from flame. Your shorba is ready. Serve in dishes with the saved onions on top.

NUTRITIONAL INFORMATION

Calories: 175 Kcal, carbohydrates:25.5g, protein 9.7g. fats: 3.8g, fibers: 3.6g cholesterol 0mg

Kale with white bean soup

- Prep time: 5 minutes.

- Cook time: 25 minutes.

- Total 30 minutes.

- Serving:4 serving

INGREDIENTS

- 2 tablespoons olive oil

- 1 small onion chopped

- 2 drained and washed cannellini beans (15 oz.)

- 4 cups chicken broth

- 2 cups water

- 2 cups kale stems, peeled and ripped into 1" pieces

- Salt and freshly ground black pepper

DIRECTION

1. Heat the oil in a 3 quart saucepan over medium-high heat until it shimmers. Cook until the onion is softened, approximately 5 minutes.
2. Meanwhile, in a small dish, mash one can of beans. Add mashed beans, broth, and water to the saucepan. Bring to a boil.
3. Stir in remaining beans (left whole) and kale. Reduce heat to low, partially cover, and cook for 20 minutes, or until kale is soft. Season with salt and pepper to taste (I use 1 teaspoon salt and 12 tsp pepper).

NUTRITIONAL INFORMATION: Serving: 2cups, Calories: 198 kcal, Carbohydrates:27g,Protein:10g Fat: 8g, Saturated Fat: 1g, Fiber: 7g, Sugar: 1g

CHAPTER 6: DESSERT RECIPE

Dark Chocolate Avocado Mousse

- Prep time: 10 mins.
- Cook time: 1 mins.
- Total: 11 minutes
- serving: 4 servings

INGREDIENTS

- 2 ripe avocados chopped
- 200 g good quality dark eating chocolate 60-75% cocoa, broken into pieces – check dairy-free if you need to
- ½ cup milk e.g. cow's, almond, coconut milk

- Two teaspoons of pure maple syrup or liquid honey are optional.

To garnish

- fresh berries or any other fruit
- grated chocolate optional

DIRECTION

1. Melt chocolate in a double boiler or in a glass bowl put over a saucepan of boiling water (be sure the water does not touch the bottom of the bowl otherwise the chocolate may burn or become gritty).
2. In a food processor, combine the avocado and melted chocolate until smooth, then add the milk.

3. Continue to combine until the mousse is extremely smooth and creamy. Taste, and if you like it sweeter, add a little honey or maple syrup; however, I believe it's sweet enough as is!

4. Spoon into serving glasses and place in the fridge for 10-15 minutes to cool. If preferred, garnish with fresh berries and more chocolate.

Nutritional information

Calories 385 Kcal, Fat 28g. Saturated Fat 12g
Carbohydrates 31g, Fiber 7g, Protein 4g Sugar 19g

Banana Nice Cream

- Prep time:10 mins.
- Total: 1 hour 10 mins
- Serving: 8 servings

INGREDIENTS

- For original banana-vanilla:
- 2 bananas, cut into 1-inch slices and solidly frozen
- 1 tablespoon almond milk
- 2 teaspoons vanilla extract
- ⅛ teaspoon salt

For chocolate:

- 2 bananas, cut into 1-inch slices and solidly frozen
- ¼ cup cocoa powder

- 2 tablespoons almond milk warmed
- ⅛ teaspoon salt

For strawberry:

- 2 bananas, cut into 1-inch slices and solidly frozen
- 1 cup strawberries stemmed, halved, and frozen solid
- 1 tablespoon almond milk
- ⅛ teaspoon salt

For peanut butter:

- 2 bananas, cut into 1-inch slices and solidly frozen
- ¼ cup creamy salted peanut butter
- 1 tablespoon almond milk
- ⅛ teaspoon cinnamon

DIRECTION

1. In a food processor, combine the bananas and the additional ingredients.

2. Blend or process until the mixture reaches the consistency of soft-serve, scraping down the sides as required and breaking up any clumped banana bits.

3. Serve immediately or store in a freezer-safe container for up to 1 month. Allow the excellent cream to remain at room temperature for a few minutes, or until it becomes scoopable, if serving from the freezer.

NUTRITIONAL INFORMATION

Calories: 121 kcal, Carbohydrates: 30g, Protein: 2g, Fat: 1g, Saturated Fat: 1g, Fiber: 4g, Sugar: 15g,

Strawberry Cheesecake Parfait

- Prep time: 15 mins
- Total 15 minutes.
- Serving: 4-6 servings

INGREDIENTS

- 1 lb fresh strawberries
- 1/4 cup granulated sugar
- 1 teaspoon lemon zest
- 1 tablespoon fresh lemon Juice
- 1.5 cups graham cracker crumbs or 1 sleeve graham crackers
- 1/4 cup unsalted butter melted
- two 8-ounce blocks cream cheese softened
- 14- ounce can sweetened condensed milk
- 1 teaspoon vanilla paste or vanilla extract

DIRECTION

1. Remove and discard the strawberry stems before cutting the strawberries into bite-sized pieces.

2. Combine the sugar, lemon zest, and lemon juice in a mixing basin. Stir everything together thoroughly, then set aside for 15 minutes.

3. In the meantime, place the graham crackers into a food processor, and pulse until ground into fine crumbs. If you don't have a food processor, use a rolling pin to smash the graham crackers.

4. In a mixing dish, combine the graham cracker crumbs and melted butter, stirring until the crumbs are coated. Place aside.

5. Whip the cream cheese, sweetened condensed milk, and vanilla paste in a large mixing basin for about a minute on medium

high speed, until the mixture is smooth and combined.

6. To make the cheesecake parfaits, spoon some of the cheesecake mixture into the bottom of a glass. Then top with a layer of buttery graham cracker crumbs.

7. Top with a layer of the macerated strawberries (discard the leftover juice), then repeat with one more layer of each. Refrigerate the parfaits for approximately an hour before serving, and enjoy!

NUTRITIONAL INFORMATION

calories: 519 kcal, carbohydrates: 77g, protein: 8g, fat: 20g, saturated fat: 12g, cholesterol: 64mg, fiber: 2g, sugar: 72g,

Dark Chocolate Avocado Truffle

- Prep time: 10 mins.
- Chill time: 30 minutes.
- Total time: 40 minutes.
- Serving: 20 servings

INGREDIENTS

- ⅔ cup mashed avocado, about 1 avocado
- 1 cup dark chocolate chips,
- Pinch of sea salt
- 2-3 Tablespoon cocoa powder

DIRECTION

1. In a food processor, add avocado and a pinch of sea salt and pulse a few times to incorporate.

2. Melt chocolate chips by placing them in a small microwave-safe bowl and microwaving for 30 seconds. Stir for another 20 seconds, or until all of the chocolate chunks have melted. (You can also do this with a double boilers

3. Pour melted chocolate into the food processor with the avocado and pulse until mixture is completely combined and avocado is no longer visible. If you don't have a food processor, use a fork to mash the avocado and blend it with the chocolate until smooth and lump-free.

4. Place the truffle mixture in the refrigerator for 30 minutes to cool.

5. Remove the mixture from the fridge once it has firmed up a little and begin making the truffles. Roll the mixture into a 1-inch ball using a tablespoon or tiny cookie scoop. You should get about 20 truffles.

6. Fill a small basin halfway with cocoa powder and roll each truffle in it until completely covered. Place on a piece of parchment paper. Refrigerate until ready to serve.

NUTRITIONAL INFORMATION

Serving: 1 truffle | Calories: 35 kcal | Carbohydrates: 4g | Protein: 1g | Fat: 3g | Saturated Fat: 1g | Cholesterol: 2mg | Fiber: 2g

Baked Apple Crumble

- Prep time: 15 minutes.
- Cook time:40 minutes.
- Total time: 55 minutes
- serving:4-6 servings

INGREDIENTS

APPLES FILLING

- 2 pound / 1 kilogram Granny Smith apples (green apples), peeled
- 1 tbsp flour , plain / all-purpose
- 1/2 cup white sugar (sub brown sugar)
- 2 tbsp lemon juice (or water)
- 1/2 tsp ground cinnamon

TOPPING

- 1 cup rolled oats or oatmeal (rapid cooking is OK)
- 1 cup flour , plain / all-purpose
- 1 cup (loosely packed) brown sugar (sub white sugar)
- 1/2 tsp baking powder
- 1 tsp cinnamon powder
- 125g / 1/2 cup melted unsalted butter
- Pinch of salt

TO SERVE

- Vanilla ice cream

DIRECTION

1. Preheat the oven to 180°C / 350°F (both fan and standard).

2. Peel apples and cut into 1.5cm/ 1/2" cubes.

3. Apple filling – Place apples in a bowl. Sprinkle flour, sugar, and cinnamon, and then drizzle with lemon juice. Toss, then spread out evenly in a 1.5 liter/1.5 quart baking dish.

4. Place the crumble topping over top. In a bowl, combine the topping ingredients. Mix until clumps form, similar to wet sand (as seen in the video). Spread over the apples, crushing with your fingers if necessary to get a crumbly topping.

5. 30 to 40 minutes, or until golden brown. Remove from the oven, cover loosely with foil to keep warm, and set aside for 10 minutes before serving (this allows the apple syrup to thicken somewhat).

6. Serve warm with vanilla ice cream!

Nutritional information

Calories:378 Kcal, Total fats : 12.6g, protein 3.6g, carbohydrates 66.1g, fiber 4.5g, sugar 42.1g

Banana Bread with Walnuts and Cinnamon

- Prep time: 10 mins
- cook time:
- 1 hour total: 1 hour 10 mins.
- serving: 12 slices

INGREDIENTS

- For the banana nut bread
- 2 cups all-purpose flour
- 1 1/2 teaspoons baking soda
- 1 teaspoon ground cinnamon
- 1 pinch salt
- 4 medium ripe bananas,mashed
- 1 cup granulated sugar
- 1/2 cup unsalted butter softened

- 2 large eggs
- 1 teaspoon vanilla extract
- 1 cup coarsely chopped walnuts, plus more for topping
- 1 tablespoon turbinado sugar, for topping
- For the sweetened condensed milk glaze
- 1/3 cups powdered sugar
- 1/3 cup sweetened condensed milk

DIRECTION

1. For the banana nut bread
2. Preheat the oven to 350°F. Set aside one big nonstick loaf pan that has been sprayed with cooking spray or brushed with butter. (I used a Wilton 9.25 x 5.25-inch pan.)
3. Combine the flour, baking soda, cinnamon, and salt in a medium mixing basin. Whisk together until combined.

4.   In a large mixing bowl, add the mashed bananas, sugar, butter, eggs, and vanilla extract. Whisk together until combined.

5.   Stir the flour mixture into the banana mixture with a wooden spoon until mixed. Fold in the chopped walnuts into the batter.

6.   Pour the batter into the prepared loaf pan. For an added crunch, top with more chopped walnuts and turbinado sugar.

7.   Bake the loaf for 60-70 minutes, or until a toothpick inserted into the center comes out clean.

8.   Remove from the oven and let the banana bread cool for 10 minutes. Then, take the banana bread from the loaf pan and cool entirely on a plate or wire rack. Top with sweetened condensed milk glaze if desired.

For the sweetened condensed milk glaze

1. Combine confectioners' sugar and sweetened condensed milk in a small mixing dish. Whisk until there are no more lumps and the mixture is fully smooth. Pour on banana nut bread and enjoy!

NUTRITIONAL INFORMATION: Serving: 1 slice with glaze Calories: 375 kcal (19%) Carbohydrates: 54g(18%) Protein: 6g (12%) Fat: 16g Fiber: 4g (16%) Sugar: 32g (36%) Cholesterol: 54mg

Mango Coconut Smoothie with Spinach and Berries

- Prep time: 5 mins,

- total time: 5 mins.

- serving:1 serving

INGREDIENTS

- 50 g baby spinach

- 180 g mango, cut into medium-sized chunks

- 2 tbsps coconut cream

- 5 g peeled and finely chopped ginger root (about 14 inch)

- 120 ml cold water

- toppings: coconut flakes, extra mango chunks, blueberry

DIRECTION

1. Add all the ingredients to the blender and blend until smooth. If it's too thick, add a little more water and mix until smooth. Serve with your favorite toppings.

Substitutions and Alteration

1. To make the smoothie sweeter: add honey, agave nectar or sweetener of choice.
2. To make it less sweet: add a little water or ice.
3. Other bases: you can substitute the water for coconut water (for added coconuttiness), coconut milk (for added richness) or juice (for added sweetness).

NUTRITIONAL INFORMATION

Serving: 1g | Calories: 414 kcal | Carbohydrates: 57g | Protein: 42g | Fat: 5g | Fiber: 6g | Sugar: 35g | Cholesterol: 123mg

Pumpkin Pie smoothie

- Prep time: 5 mins,
- total time: 5 mins.
- serving:2 servings

INGREDIENTS

- 1 large banana sliced and frozen
- 1/2 cup almond milk, unsweetened Greek yogurt (I chose Kite Hill) - any paleo-friendly yogurt would do.
- 1/2 cup pureed pumpkin
- 2 tablespoons of maple syrup or 2 pitted medjool dates
- Add 1/2 cup unsweetened vanilla almond milk for a thinner smoothie.
- 1 teaspoon vanilla extract
- 1/4 teaspoon ground cinnamon

- 1/2 teaspoon pumpkin pie spice
- 1/2-1 cup ice cubes optional
- 1 scoop vanilla collagen protein or vegan vanilla protein,optional

for a smoothie bowl (makes 1 large):

- Reduce the milk to 1/3 cup
- Do not add ice

DIRECTION

1. Blend all of the ingredients in a high-speed blender, such as a Vitamix, until smooth and creamy.
2. .For a regular smoothie, pour into glasses and top with a little cinnamon or coconut whipped cream to serve. For a smoothie bowl, pour into a bowl and add desired

toppings like grain free granola, pumpkin seeds, almond butter, sliced bananas and a drizzle of maple syrup. Enjoy!

NUTRITIONAL INFORMATION

Calories: 184 kcal, Carbohydrates: 39g, Protein: 7g,Fat: 1g, Cholesterol: 3mg, Fiber : 5g, Sugar: 27g

No-Bake Peanut Butter Oatmeal Cookies

- Prep time: 10 minutes
- Cook time: 5 minutes
- Additional time: 1 hour
- Total time: 1 hour 15 minutes
- Serving: 34 cookies

INGREDIENTS

- 1 & 1/2 cups (300g) firmly packed light or dark brown sugar
- 1/2 cup (113g) unsalted butter
- 1/2 cup (118ml) milk
- 1 cup (255g) creamy peanut butter
- 1 teaspoon vanilla extract
- 1 teaspoon salt

- 3 cups (297g) old-fashioned rolled oats

DIRECTION

1. Line baking sheets with parchment paper. Set aside.
2. Brown sugar, milk, and butter should all be combined in a big pot. Cook, tossing regularly, over medium heat until butter melts.
3. Increase the heat to medium-high, and bring to a boil. Boil for 1 minute.
4. Remove from the heat and mix in the peanut butter, vanilla extract, and salt. Stir until smooth.
5. Stir in the oats.
6. Drop the cookies by tablespoonfuls onto the prepared pans, allowing approximately an inch between each.

7. Refrigerate 1 hour, or until set

NUTRITIONAL INFORMATION

Calories:4 Kcal, carbohydrates:1g, total fats:2g, protein:4g, sugar:2g cholesterol: 5mg

lentil mint fudge

- Prep time:20 mins

- cook time: 15 mins

- total: 35 minutes

- serving:36 servings

INGREDIENTS

- 1/3 cup sunflower seeds, toasted

- 1/2 cup coconut flakes, toasted

- 1 cup washed and drained cooked or canned green lentils

- 3 tablespoon raw cacao powder

- 3 tablespoons raw honey (or a few drops Stevia if vegan)

- 3 tablespoons coconut oil

- 1/2 teaspoon peppermint extract

- 1/2 cup walnuts, chopped

DIRECTION

1. In a food processor, combine the seeds, flakes, lentils, cacao, and honey and pulse until smooth, scraping down the sides once or twice.

2. Melt the coconut oil in a small glass bowl in the microwave for a few seconds, until a liquid develops. Combine it with the peppermint and walnuts in the lentil mixture. Stir until everything is mixed.

3. Line a small pyrex dish with parchment paper and equally distribute the ingredients around both edges. Refrigerate for at least 3 hours before serving, and store any leftovers in the refrigerator.

NUTRITIONAL INFORMATION

Calories: 101 kcal (5%,), Carbohydrates: 14g (5%),
Protein: 1g (2%) Fat: 5g (8%), Fiber: 0.02g Sugar:
13g (14%)

CHAPTER 7: SALAD RECIPE

Caprese Salad with Avocado

- Prep time: 5 minutes.
- Total time: 5 minutes.
- Serving:6 servings

INGREDIENTS

- 3 tablespoons balsamic vinegar
- 2 tablespoons extra-virgin olive oil
- ½ teaspoon salt
- ½ teaspoon ground pepper
- 1 ½ cups multi colored cherry tomatoes, halved
- 2 ripe avocados, diced
- 4 ounces small fresh mozzarella balls
- 1 tablespoon drained capers (optional)

- ½ cup lightly packed fresh basil leaves

DIRECTIONS

1. Mix the vinegar, oil, salt, and pepper in a small basin. In a large bowl, combine tomatoes, avocados, mozzarella, and capers, if using. Toss to coat after adding the dressing and basil.

NUTRITIONAL INFORMATION

Calories 218 Kcal ,Total Carbohydrate 9g, Dietary Fiber 5g, Total Sugars 3g, Total Fat 19g, cholesterol 13mg, protein 5g

Citrus Spinach Salad

- Prep time:15 minutes

- total time: 15 minutes.

- Serving:12 servings

INGREDIENTS

- 3 tablespoons honey

- 2 tablespoons lime juice

- 1 teaspoon grated lime zest

- 1/8 to 1/4 teaspoon ground nutmeg

- 1/3 cup canola oil

- 10 cups torn fresh spinach

- 3 medium navel oranges, peeled and sectioned

- 2 medium pink grapefruit, peeled and sectioned

DIRECTION

1. In a blender, join the honey, lime juice, lime zing and nutmeg; cover and cycle until

mixed. While handling, bit by bit add oil in a constant flow until dressing is thickened.

2. In an enormous plate of mixed greens bowl, consolidate the spinach, oranges and grapefruit.Drizzle with dressing; toss to coat. Top with onion. Serve immediately.

NUTRITIONAL INFORMATION

1 serving: 109 calories, 6g fat (1g saturated fat), 0 cholesterol, 21mg, carbohydrate (11g sugars, 2g fiber), 1g protein

Tomato Basil Quinoa Salad

- Prep time: 30 minutes.

- Cook time: 2 hours.

- Total time: 2 hours 30 minutes

- serving:4 servings

INGREDIENTS

- 2 cups quinoa, rinsed and drained

- 2 cloves garlic, peeled and minced

- 4 cups water

- Kosher salt

- 2 tablespoons extra-virgin olive oil

- 10-12 big basil leaves, thinly sliced

- 1/2 pound cherry tomatoes, halved

- Freshly ground black pepper

DIRECTIONS

1. The quinoa, garlic, water, and 1/2 teaspoon kosher salt should all be brought to a rolling

boil in a medium saucepan over high heat, stirring from time to time.

2. Reduce the heat to low, and simmer until the quinoa has entirely absorbed the water, about 15 minutes. Remove from the heat and set aside. After the quinoa has cooled for 15 minutes, chill in the cooler for something like 2 hours.

3. In a serving bowl, throw the chilled quinoa with the olive oil, basil, tomatoes, and salt and pepper to taste. Act as a serving of mixed greens or a side.

NUTRITIONAL INFORMATION

Calories 248 Kcal Total Carbohydrate 30g, Dietary Fiber 5g, Total Sugars 8g, Total Fat 12g, protein 6g

Greek Farro Salad

- Prep time: 15 minutes
- Cook time: 25 minutes
- Total time :40 minutes
- Serving: 4 servings

INGREDIENTS

Salad

- 1 cup dried farro, rinsed
- 5 cups lightly packed arugula (if it's not 5 cups delicately stuffed arugula (in the event that it's not child arugula, you should give it a couple of cleaves to break it into more modest pieces)
- 1 can chickpeas, washed and depleted (or 1 ½ cups cooked chickpeas))
- 1 large cucumber (about ¾ pound), seeded and chopped (to yield about 1 ½ cup chopped cucumber)

- 1 cup hacked broiled red chime pepper, custom made or jolted
- 20 kalamata olives, cut into slim rounds (about ½ cup)
- ½ cup feta cheese, crumbled
- ½ cup chopped flat-leaf parsley
- ¼ teaspoon salt

Dressing

- ⅓ cup olive oil
- 2 to 3 tablespoons new lemon juice, to taste
- 2 teaspoons honey or maple syrup
- 2 garlic cloves, pressed
- ½ teaspoon dried oregano
- ½ teaspoon salt
- ¼ teaspoon red pepper flakes
- Freshly ground black pepper, to taste

DIRECTION

1. To cook the farro: In a medium pot, join the flushed farro with no less than three cups of water (enough water to cover the farro by several inches).

2. Heat the water to the point of boiling, then diminish intensity to a delicate stew. Cook, mixing at times, until the farro is delicate to the chomp yet enjoyably chewy (pearled farro will require about 15 minutes; natural farro will require 25 to 40 minutes).

3. Channel off the overabundant water and return the farro to the pot. Mix in ¼ teaspoon salt and a little sprinkle of the dressing. Put away for only a couple of moments to cool.

4. In the meantime, in a huge serving bowl, join the arugula, chickpeas, cucumber, peppers, olives and parsley.

5. In a fluid estimating cup or little bowl, whisk together the olive oil, lemon juice, honey,

garlic, oregano, salt, red pepper chips and pepper until emulsified.

6. Pour the remaining dressing over the heated farro in the serving basin. Toss to combine. Add the feta, throw once more, and season to taste with extra salt and pepper.

NUTRITIONAL INFORMATION

Calories: 571Kcal, total fats : 30.2g, carbohydrates: 61.3 g, protein; 15.6g, sugar:7.1g, fiber: 13.8g, cholesterol:16.7mg

Mango tango spinach salad

- Prep time:20 mins
- Total time: 20 mins
- Serving:8 servings

INGREDIENTS

- 2 mangos cubed
- 2 avocados cubed
- 4 tomatoes chunked
- 1/4 C. finely chopped green onions
- 4 C. chopped fresh spinach
- 1/4 C. finely chopped cucumbers
- 1 C. raspberry vinaigrette dressing
- 1/2 C. Mozzarella cheese shredded
- 1/4 C. sliced almonds
- 1/4 C. chopped fresh cilantro

DIRECTIONS

1. In a huge serving bowl join mangos, avocados, tomatoes, onion, spinach, cucumbers, and dressing, and daintily throw.

2. Sprinkle cheddar, almonds, and cilantro equally over top of salad preceding serving. Yet again preceding serving delicately throw and serve.

NUTRITIONAL INFORMATION

Calories: 227.8kcal Carbohydrates: 54.9g Protein: 4.3g Fat:1.9g Fiber: 7.9g Sugar: 46.3g

Lentil Salad

- Prep time: 5 mins
- Cook time: 15 mins
- Total time: 20 mins
- Serving:6 servings

INGREDIENTS

For the salad:

- One cup of raw green lentils, thoroughly rinsed and inspected
- 3 cups water (or vegetable broth)
- 1 bay leaf
- 1 English cucumber, finely diced
- 1 stemmed, seeded, and finely sliced red bell pepper
- 1/2 small red onion, finely diced
- 1/4 cup chopped Italian parsley
- 1/4 cup chopped fresh mint leaves
- 1/3 cup crumbled feta cheese,optional

For the dressing:

- 1/4 cup olive oil

- 2 teaspoons lemon zest

- 2 tablespoons fresh lemon juice

- 1 teaspoon Dijon mustard

- 1 teaspoon honey or pure maple syrup

- 1 clove garlic, minced

- Kosher salt and black pepper, to taste

DIRECTIONS

1. Combine the lentils, water or broth, and bay leaf in a large pot. Bring to a boil over medium-high heat, then reduce to a low heat and simmer for 15 to 20 minutes, or until the lentils are cooked but slightly hard. Overcooking will result in mushy lentils.

2. While the lentils are cooking, make the dressing. Whisk together the olive oil, lemon zest, lemon juice, Dijon mustard, honey or

maple syrup, garlic, salt, and pepper in a small bowl or jar. Place aside.

3. When the lentils are done cooking, rinse them in a colander. Discard the bay leaf. Rinse quickly with cold water. Transfer to a large bowl.

4. Add the cucumber, mint, parsley, red pepper, red onion, and, if using, feta cheese to the bowl. Stir. Toss with the dressing until fully mixed. Serve immediately or set aside for 30 minutes to allow the flavors to blend.

NUTRITIONAL INFORMATION

Calories: 217 kcal, Carbohydrates: 25g, Protein: 10g, Fat: 9g, Fiber: 11g, Sugar: 4g,

Protein-Packed Chicken Arugula Salad

- Prep time: 15 minutes
- Cook time: 15 minutes
- Total: 30 minutes
- Serving:4 servings

INGREDIENTS

- 12 cups of cleaned and dried arugula leaves
- 1 pint cherry tomatoes, each cut in half
- 1 15-ounce can washed and drained white beans
- 4 tablespoons olive oil, divided
- 3 cloves garlic, minced
- 1 pound chicken tenders, peeled and cut into bite-size pieces
- Salt and freshly ground black pepper
- 3 tablespoons balsamic vinegar
- 2 1/2 teaspoons grainy mustard

- 2 ounces grated Asiago cheese (approximately 1/2 cup)

DIRECTIONS

1. In a large mixing bowl, combine arugula, cherry tomatoes, and white beans.

2. 1 1/2 teaspoons olive oil, heated in a medium nonstick skillet over medium heat. Add the garlic, chicken tenders, and a few pinches of salt and pepper; heat until the chicken is moist and barely cooked through, about 5 minutes. Add to salad.

3. In a small dish, combine the remaining 2 1/2 tablespoons olive oil, vinegar, and mustard. Coat the salad by tossing it with the dressing.

4. Arrange salad on four dinner plates and top with Asiago cheese.

NUTRITIONAL INFORMATION

Serves 4; Nutritional information per serving (2 1/2 cups with 1/4 pound chicken tenders): 445 calories, 32% fat (16 g), 31% carbohydrate (34 g), 37% protein (41 g), 7 g fiber,

Steak & Asparagus Salad

- Prep time:20 minutes.

- Cook time: 10 minutes

- Total time: 30 minutes

- Serving: 2 serving

INGREDIENTS

- 3 tablespoons garlic oil

- 2 tablespoons fresh lemon juice

- To taste, season with salt and freshly ground black pepper.

- 12 cups mixed spring greens

- 1 pound asparagus, tough ends snapped off

- 4 large eggs

- 1 pound raw flank steak

- 2 cloves garlic

- 1 tablespoon soy sauce

- Four pieces of toasted whole-grain sandwich bread, sliced into tiny squares

- 8 teaspoons grated Parmesan cheese

DIRECTIONS

1. Preheat a grill or broiler to medium. To make the salad dressing, whisk together the lemon juice and garlic oil until well blended. After adding salt and pepper to taste, reserve.

2. In a large salad dish, combine mixed spring greens. Bring a big skillet of water to a boil by filling it halfway. When the asparagus is soft but still crisp, add it and simmer for 6 minutes. Using a slotted spoon, remove spears and set aside to cool.

3. Return the water in the same skillet to a boil. Poach eggs by cracking each egg open and carefully putting it into the water. Cook for 3 to 6 minutes over medium-low heat, occasionally spooning water over the yolks to

assist them cook (yolks should be soft-cooked when done).

4. Garlic, soy sauce, and several pinches of salt and pepper should be applied to both sides of the flank steak. Put the meat on the broiler pan or grill. Cook for 4 minutes, then flip and cook for another 4 minutes, or until the steak, when cut, is pink in the middle. Place meat on chopping board and allow to rest.

5. Cut the chilled asparagus into 1-inch pieces and add it to the salad dish with the bread squares. Half of the dressing should be tossed with the salad ingredients.

6. Divide salad among four shallow salad bowls. Place a poached egg over greens. Cut the flank steak into thin slices on the diagonal, then place the steak pieces around each egg. To serve, drizzle salads with steak juices and the remaining dressing, then top with Parmesan cheese.

NUTRITIONAL INFORMATION

Serves 4; Nutritional information per serving (3 cups salad, 1 egg, 1 slice whole-grain toast, 3 ounces flank steak, and 2 teaspoons Parmesan cheese): 473 calories, 49% fat (26 g), 20% carbohydrate (24 g), 31% protein (37 g), 6 g fiber

Pork and Spinach Salad

- Prep time: 45 minutes

- Cook time: 2 hours

- Total time: 2 hours 45 minutes

- Serving:6 servings

INGREDIENTS

- 1 pound pork tenderloin, fat trimmed

- 2 teaspoons olive oil

- 1 teaspoon ground cumin

- 1 teaspoon ground coriander

- To taste, season with salt and freshly ground black pepper.

- 1/2 cup whole-wheat couscous

- 6 whole dried figs, chopped

- 1 cup red grapes, cut in half

- 2 ounces aged pasteurized goat cheese, crumbled

- 1/4 cup honey

- 1/3 cup balsamic vinegar

- 12 cups spinach leaves, washed

DIRECTIONS

1. Heat grill to medium or oven to 375° F.

2. Brush tenderloin with olive oil, then season with cumin, coriander, and salt and pepper to taste.

3. Grill or bake tenderloin for 8 minutes on one side on a foil-lined baking sheet. Cook for 7 to 8 minutes more, or until rosy yet cooked through.

4. Remove the tenderloin from the grill or oven and let aside for 1 minute before slicing into 1/2-inch thick slices.

5. In a medium saucepan, bring 1 cup of water to a boil while the pork cooks. Once the couscous is added, remove from the fire. After covering the pan, give the couscous ten minutes to rest. Transfer the couscous to a medium mixing bowl and fluff with a fork. When cool, add figs, grapes, and goat cheese.

6. In a small basin, whisk together the honey and balsamic vinegar until the honey dissolves. Pour half of the dressing over the couscous and toss lightly to combine. Season with salt and pepper.

7. Divide spinach among four large plates. Place a piece of the couscous mixture on top, followed by the pork slices. Drizzle with remaining dressing.

NUTRITIONAL INFORMATION

517 calories, 21% fat (12 g), 54% carbohydrate (70 g), 25% protein (32 g), 9 g fiber,

Zupas Copycat Strawberry Harvest Salad

- Prep time: 10 minutes.
- Total time: 10 minutes.
- Serving: 4 servings

INGREDIENTS

Pureed Strawberry Vinaigrette

- 2 tbsp. olive oil
- 2 tbsp. white vinegar
- 1 1/2 c. fresh strawberries
- 1/3 c. fresh squeezed lemon juice
- 2 tablespoons real maple syrup

Brown Sugar Pecans

- 1/4 c. brown sugar
- 1/4 c. butter
- 2 c. chopped pecans or pecan pieces

Additional Salad Ingredients

- baby spinach or arugula

- green leaf or romaine lettuce, chopped

- shredded or diced rotisserie chicken breast (or cook your own chicken)

- fresh strawberries, quartered

- grated Fontina cheese

- apples, thinly sliced

- salt and pepper, to taste

- red onions, diced fine(optional)

DIRECTION

Pureed Strawberry Vinaigrette

- Combine vinaigrette ingredients in a blender. Puree until smooth. Mix well before serving. Keep in an airtight jar in the refrigerator.

Brown Sugar Pecans

- Place butter into a small saucepan and melt on medium-low heat.

- Add brown sugar and mix until blended. Then add pecans and cook until brown sugar starts to caramelize. Watch carefully and stir consistently so they don't burn. Reduce the heat and whisk continuously if you smell burn.Once bubbling, they are starting to caramelize. Give them a minute or two to bubble (without burning).

- Place onto a cooling rack or parchment paper.

Salad

- The number of salad ingredients should be adjusted based on the number of guests.

- Begin assembling salad by mixing lettuce and spinach. Top with plenty of chicken and strawberries. Then add in sliced apples and pecans. Top with grated Fontina cheese and if using, diced red onions, and a little fresh cracked pepper and salt.

- Just before serving, top with strawberry vinaigrette. Enjoy!

NUTRITIONAL INFORMATION

Serving: 1g, Calories: 339kcal, Carbohydrates: 30g, Protein: 17g, Fat: 18g,Fiber: 5g, Sugar: 24g,Cholesterol: 47mg,

CHAPTER 8:
VEGETARIAN RECIPE

Eggplant Parmesan

- Prep time:20 minutes
- Cook time: 40 minutes
- Total time: 1hour
- Serving: 6-8 servings
- Course: Dinner

INGREDIENTS

- 2 huge eggplant circles, 14-inch thick
- 2 eggs, beaten
- ¼ cup almond milk
- 1½ cups panko breadcrumbs
- 1¼ cup grated Parmesan cheese, divided
- 2 teaspoons oregano
- 2 tablespoons fresh thyme

- ½ teaspoon red pepper flakes

- ½ teaspoon sea salt, more for sprinkling

- Freshly ground black pepper

- Extra-virgin olive oil, for drizzling

- 28 ounces Marinara Sauce

- 2 large balls fresh mozzarella, thinly sliced

- ⅓ cup fresh basil leaves

DIRECTION

1. Preheat the oven to 400 degrees Fahrenheit and prepare two baking pans with parchment paper.

2. Combine the panko, 1 cup Parmesan cheese, oregano, thyme, red pepper flakes, salt, and several grinds of pepper in another medium-sized shallow dish.

3. Dip the eggplant slices into the egg mixture and then into the panko mixture. Place onto the baking sheets, drizzle with olive oil, and

bake for 18 minutes or until tender and golden brown.

4. Spread 12 cup marinara in an 8x12 or 9x13-inch baking dish, put half the eggplant, and top with 1 cup marinara and half the mozzarella. Repeat with the remaining eggplant, marinara, and mozzarella until all of the ingredients are used. Drizzle with olive oil and a couple more pinches of sea salt before topping with the remaining 14 cup Parmesan cheese. Bake for 20 minutes, or until the cheese is melted and bubbling. Preheat the oven to broil for 2 to 4 minutes, or until the cheese is browned and bubbling.

5. Remove from the oven and sprinkle with fresh basil.

NUTRITIONAL INFORMATION

Calories:403 Kcal, carbohydrates:36.6g, protein:25.4g, fats:17.5g, sugar 6.7g, cholesterol:109.1mg

Broccoli and Cheddar Quiche

- Prep time:30 minutes
- Cook time: 1 hour
- Total time: 1 hour 30 minutes
- Serving:8 servings
- Course: Breakfast & brunch

INGREDIENTS

- All-purpose flour, for rolling
- 1 homemade or store-bought single-crust pie dough
- 1 tablespoon unsalted butter
- 2 cups medium yellow onion chopped (from 1 big onion)
- Coarse salt and ground pepper
- 6 large eggs
- ¾ cup heavy cream

- ¾ pound broccoli florets, steamed until crisp-tender

- 1 cup grated sharp cheddar (4 ounces)

DIRECTION

Preheat oven and roll out pie dough:

- Preheat the oven to 375 degrees. Roll out the dough to a 12-inch circular on a lightly floured work surface

Fit dough into pie plate:

- Fold overhang under and crimp edge of a 9-inch pie pan.

Add parchment paper and pie weights:

- Cover the dough with parchment paper and fill with pie weights or dry beans

Blind bake crust:

- Bake until the edge is dry and light golden, about 20 minutes. Remove parchment and weights.

Melt butter and cook onion:

- Meanwhile, melt the butter in a large pan over medium-high heat. Season with salt and pepper and sauté until the onion is light golden, 8 to 10 minutes.

Whisk eggs and cream together:

- Beat the eggs and cream together in a medium-sized

.Add onion, broccoli, and cheese:

- Add onion, broccoli florets, and cheese and season with 1/2 teaspoon salt and 1/4 teaspoon pepper.

Whisk and pour into crust:

- Whisk to combine, pour into the crucru

Bake:

- Bake for 40 to 45 minutes, or until the quiche's center is barely set. Serve warm or at room temperature.

NUTRITIONAL INFORMATION

calories 282 Kcal Total Fat 19g,Total Carbohydrate 18g,Dietary Fiber 2g,Total Sugars 2g, protein 11g, cholesterol 138 mg

Spinach and Ricotta Stuffed Shells

- Prep time: 15 minutes.

- Time to cook: 35 minutes;

- total time: 50 minutes.

- Serving:4 servings

- Course: Dinner

INGREDIENTS

- 16 large pasta shells (Cook a few extra shells in case they break while the pasta cooks.)

- 1–1/2 tbsp olive oil

- 2 tsp fresh garlic, minced

- 4 cups (packed) fresh spinach leaves, roughly-chopped

- 12 oz skim-milk ricotta cheese

- 1 cup shredded skim-milk mozzarella cheese

- 1/2 cup grated Parmesan cheese, plus additional for serving

- 1 large egg

- 1 tbsp fresh basil, finely chopped

- 1 tsp kosher salt

- 1/2 tsp freshly-ground black pepper

- 1–1/4 cups marinara sauce

DIRECTION

1. Preheat the oven to 375 degrees F. Cook the pasta until it is al dente, as directed on the box. Set aside after draining.

2. Meanwhile, in a large pan over medium-high heat, heat the olive oil. When the oil begins to shimmer, add the garlic and sauté for a minute or two, or until it begins to brown. Cook, stirring periodically, until the spinach leaves begin to wilt but remain brilliant green, about 3 to 4 minutes. The spinach should be cut in half. After turning off the heat, remove the pan and let it cool.

3. In a mixing bowl, combine the spinach, ricotta, mozzarella, Parmesan, egg, basil, and

salt & pepper to taste. Pour 1/2 cup of the marinara sauce into the bottom of a shallow 8-inch by 8-inch baking dish. Place each pasta shell in the baking dish and fill with a liberal quantity of the spinach and ricotta mixture.

4. Cover with the remaining sauce and bake for 25 minutes, covered with aluminum foil. Remove the cover and bake for another 10-15 minutes, or until the top begins to brown and the sauce begins to boil. Serve warm with a dusting of Parmesan.

NUTRITIONAL INFORMATION

Serving:407gCalories:798cal(40%)

Carbohydrates:69g(23%)Protein:43g(86%)

Fat:39g(60%)Cholesterol:145mg(48%)   Fiber:8g

(33%)Sugar:14g (16%)

Quinoa & vegetable stuffed Portobello Mushroom

- Prep time: 5 minutes.

- Cook time: 25 minutes

- Total time: 30 minutes.

- Serving: 4 servings

- course: Entree

INGREDIENTS

FILLINGS

- 1 teaspoon avocado, coconut, or water

- 1/2 cup uncooked quinoa* (or 1 1/4 cup (230 g) cooked quinoa as original recipe is written // adjust if altering batch size)

- 1 Tbsp melted coconut oil or avocado oil

- 1 1/2 cups organic diced sweet potatoes (or butternut squash)

- 1 cup sliced bell pepper (red is my favorite)

- 1 cup chopped red cabbage

- 1 tsp ground cumin (divided)
- 1 tsp chili powder (or smoked paprika // divided)
- 1/2 tsp sea salt (divided)
- 1/2 cup cooked black beans(cooking/canning liquid drained)

MUSHROOMS

- 4 large portobello mushrooms*(stems removed, wiped clean)
- 1-2 Tbsp avocado or melted coconut oil (or sub water or vegetable broth)
- 2 Tbsp balsamic vinegar
- 1 Tbsp lime juice
- 1/2 tsp ground cumin (divided)
- 1/4 tsp chili powder or smoked paprika (divided)
- 1/4 tsp sea salt
- 1 Tbsp lime juice

FOR SERVING optional

- Magic Green Sauce
- Easy Red Salsa
- Limes
- Cilantro

DIRECTION

1. Preheat the oven to 400°F (204°C) and prepare a rimmed baking sheet or a big baking dish.(Or, if grilling, heat grill.)

2. Start by heating a medium pot over medium heat if you don't have any cooked quinoa on hand. Once hot, add avocado oil or coconut oil or water (1 tsp as original recipe is written) and rinsed and drained quinoa (1/2 cup as original recipe is written). To toast, sauté for 1-2 minutes, stirring often. Then add 1 cup water and a pinch of salt (amounts as given in the original recipe // modify if batch size changes).

3. Bring to a boil over medium-high heat. Then reduce heat to simmer and cook until liquid has mostly absorbed and the quinoa is tender (~15-18 minutes). Drain off any excess liquid if needed. Then, turn off the heat and leave it uncovered to allow any extra moisture to evaporate.

4. Meanwhile, season the mushrooms with oil (or water or vegetable broth), balsamic vinegar, lime juice, cumin, chili powder, and sea salt in a shallow baking or serving dish. To mix, flip/toss and set away to marinade.

5. Then, in a big pan over medium heat, prepare the veggies. Once heated, add oil or water (1 Tbsp (15 ml) as specified in the original recipe // modify if batch size changes), sweet potatoes, and bell pepper. Cook for 3-5 minutes (covered), or until slightly browned.

6. Add cabbage, 1/2 tsp cumin, 1/2 tsp chili powder, and 1/4 tsp sea salt (amounts as

original recipe is written // adjust if altering batch size) and sauté for another 3-5 minutes, or until all veggies (particularly the potato) are soft and golden brown. Place aside.

7. Set aside the veggies from the skillet in a large mixing basin. Then, in the same skillet over medium heat, brown and soften the mushrooms for 2 minutes on both sides. For the last minute, cover and softly steam. Then transfer to a baking sheet face up and set aside.

8. To the mixing bowl with the vegetables, add cooked quinoa, drained black beans, remaining 1/2 tsp cumin, 1/2 tsp chili powder, 1/4 tsp sea salt (amounts as original recipe is written // adjust if batch size changes), and lime juice and stir to blend.

9. Divide the filling evenly among the mushrooms (some may overflow, which is acceptable). Bake at 400 degrees (or on the

grill, covered) for about 5 minutes or until mushrooms and toppings are hot and slightly browned.

10. Enjoy immediately as is or with a sauce of choice (optional // I think the magic green sauce goes awesome with this recipe!). Refrigerate leftovers separately from sauce(s) for 3-4 days, covered. Reheat until hot in a 350°F (176°C) oven or microwave.

NUTRITIONAL INFORMATION

Nutrition (1 of 4 servings)

Serving: 1 serving   Calories: 305 Carbohydrates: 50.5 g Protein: 9.2 g Fat: 8.5g, Cholesterol: 0 mg Fiber: 10 g Sugar: 11.7 g

Cauliflower and Chickpea Curry

- Prep time: 10 minutes
- Cook time: 20 minutes.
- Total time: 30 minutes.
- Serving:4 servings.
- Course: Dinner

DIRECTION

- 4 tbsp vegetable oil
- 1 tbsp ginger finely grated
- 3 large garlic cloves minced.
- 1 large onion chopped (brown, white, yellow)
- 3 tsp coriander powder
- 1/4 tsp turmeric powder
- 1 tsp cumin powder
- 2 tsp paprika
- 1 1/2 cups chicken stock

- 800 g crushed tomato (28 oz can) 300 g packed cauliflower tiny florets (1 small / 1/2 big cauliflower)
- 400 g / 14 oz drained chickpeas Salt
- Salt
- 1 tsp sugar - optional
- 3/4 cup frozen peas 75g
- 3 tsp garam masala powder
- 1/4 cup coriander / cilantro leaves chopped
- Yogurt to serve (highly recommended)

DIRECTION

1. In a big deep skillet or saucepan, heat the oil over medium high heat. Cook for 1 minute after adding the garlic and ginger. Cook for 6 to 8 minutes, or until brown and caramelized

2. .Add coriander, turmeric, cumin and paprika. Cook for 1 minute.

3. Add chicken stock and tomato. Stir everything together, bring to a simmer, and cook for 5 minutes.

4. Add cauliflower and chickpeas. Cook for 15 minutes, or until the cauliflower softens and the sauce thickens. Put the lid on if the sauce is thickening too soon. Adjust the salt to taste, and if using, add the sugar.

5. Add peas and garam masala. Cook for 2 minutes before removing from heat. Stir through most of the coriander.

6. Serve the stew over basmati rice or plain white rice, topped with the saved coriander and yogurt on the side.

NUTRITION INFORMATION:

Serving:552g   Calories:344   cal   (17%.)
Carbohydrates:44.1g (15%)   Protein:10.7g (21%)
Fat:15.8g (24%)   Fiber:11.6g (48%.)   Sugar:11.5g (13%)

Quinoa and kale stuffed acorn squash

- Prep time: 20 minutes.

- Cook time: 50 minutes

- total: 1 hour 10 minutes

- serving: 8 servings

- course: Entree, main course and side dish

INGREDIENTS

- 2 acorn squash, halved and seeded (each 2 1/2 to 3 lb)

- 1/4 cup olive oil

- 1 tsp each salt and freshly ground pepper

- 1/2 tsp each ground allspice and cinnamon

- 1 onion, finely chopped

- 3 cloves garlic, minced

- 2 tbsp chopped fresh sage

- 6 cups stemmed shredded kale

- 3 tbsp apple cider vinegar

- 2 tbsp maple syrup
- 2 tbsp grainy mustard
- 3 cups cooked quinoa
- 1/2 cup chopped walnuts, toasted
- 1/4 cup dried cranberries
- 2 cups (8oz) Burnett Dairy Mozzarella Shredded Cheese
- 1/4 cup chopped fresh parsley

DIRECTION

1. Preheat the oven to 425°F. Line the baking sheet with parchment paper. Brush cut sides of squash with 2 tbsp olive oil and season with half each salt and pepper, allspice and cinnamon. Place on a baking sheet lined with parchment paper and bake for 40 to 45 minutes, or until tender.

2. Meanwhile, in a large skillet, heat remaining oil over medium heat; cook onion, garlic and sage, stirring, for 3 to 5 minutes or until

onion is tender. Cook for 1 minute, or until the kale is slightly wilted. Stir in vinegar, maple syrup and mustard; stir in quinoa, walnuts and cranberries. Remove from heat; toss with 1 cup cheese and remaining salt and pepper.

3. Divide the quinoa mixture evenly among the squash halves; top with the remaining cheese. Bake for 6 to 8 minutes, or until the mixture is hot and the cheese melts. Sprinkle with parsley.

4. **Tip:** For meatier stuffed squash, add 1 cooked and crumbled Italian sausage to the stuffing or 1/3 cup cooked chopped pancetta.

   Cook the squash and create the filling a day ahead of time to save time. Allow extra time for the filling to cook through during baking.

NUTRITIONAL INFORMATION

Calories: 507 kcal | Carbohydrates: 56g | Protein: 10g | Fat: 29g | Fiber: 6g | Sugar: 13g

CHAPTER 9: SNACKS RECIPE

Edamame

- Prep time: 10 minutes,

- Cook time: 5 minutes.

- Total time:. 15 minutes

INGREDIENTS

- 1 pound frozen edamame pods (in shell)

- ½ tablespoon toasted sesame oil

- 1 small garlic clove

- 34 teaspoon kosher or fine sea salt, plus additional salt for the water

- Spicy version: 1 tablespoon chili garlic sauce (to taste)

- Optional garnish: Toasted sesame seeds

DIRECTION

1. Bring a large saucepan of water to a boil. Add one teaspoon of kosher salt and the edamame

2. Boil the edamame until bright green and tender, about 4 to 5 minutes, then drain.

3. Place the edamame in a bowl. Add the toasted sesame oil and salt, then grate the garlic clove (with a microplane) into the bowl. Toss gently until everything is uniformly coated, breaking up any garlic clumps that form. Serve heated in a serving bowl, with a smaller bowl for the discarded pods.

NUTRITIONAL INFORMATION

Calories: 139   Kcal,   carbohydrates:8.6g, protein:12.7g, fats:7.1g, Fiber: 5.4g, sugar:2.8g

Tuna Seaweed Snacks

- Prep time:15 minutes.
- Total: 15 minutes.
- Serving:2 servings

INGREDIENTS

- 1 small can tuna, in water(approx. 120 grams or 4 oz. DRAINED)
- 1.5 Tbsp mayonnaise (I used avocado oil mayo)
- 1 Persian cucumber, diced (about 1/4 English cucumber)
- 1 stalk celery, diced
- 1/4 cup green onion, diced
- 2 tsp sriracha (or to desired spiciness)
- 1/2 tsp garlic powder

- Salt + pepper, to taste

- 8 squares nori seaweed (tear huge sheets into smaller pieces or use seaweed snacks)

- Sesame seeds (optional garnish)

DIRECTION

1. Drain excess water out of canned tuna. Transfer to a large mixing basin and mash with a fork.

2. Add chopped cucumber, celery, green onion, mayo, sriracha, garlic powder, salt, and pepper to the same bowl.

3. Stir ingredients together until well combined. Adjust the ingredients to taste, making it more spicy or "mayo-y" as desired.Keep in mind that the amount of salt you use will be determined by how salty your seaweed snacks are! If you buy unsalted nori, you'll need to add more salt to the tuna combination

than if you use pre-seasoned tuna snacks. You can always add more when serving as needed!

4. When using bigger sheets of nori, cut each sheet into four pieces. Alternatively, arrange seaweed snacks on a dish and top with the tuna combination. The recipe as stated should yield around 8 "bites" or "wraps."

5. Garnish with sesame seeds and more sriracha, if desired. Eat the tuna seaweed snacks as bite-sized wraps right away.

NUTRITIONAL INFORMATION

Calories: 80 Kcal, Total Fat: 4g, Total Carbohydrate: 1g, protein: 8g, dietary Fiber: 0g, Total Sugar:1 g, cholesterol:145 mg

Fruit and nut butter sandwiches

- Prep time:10 minutes,
- total time: 10 minutes.
- Serving:1 serving

INGREDIENTS

- 2 tablespoons chunky or creamy peanut butter
- 1 tablespoon raisins
- ¼ cup chopped apple
- 1 tablespoon unsalted dry roasted peanuts
- 2 tablespoons strawberry jam
- 2 slices whole-grain bread

DIRECTIONS

1. On one side of a slice of bread, spread peanut butter and sprinkle with diced apple, raisins, and peanuts.

2. To prepare a sandwich, spread jam on the remaining slice of bread and top with fruit and nuts.

NUTRITIONAL INFORMATION

Servings Per Recipe 1 Calories 530 Kcal, carbohydrate: 70g, Protein 17g Total Fat 23g, Total Sugars 40g, Dietary Fiber 8g

Fruit And Nut Trail Mix

- Total time: 30 minutes
- serving: 7 servings

INGREDIENTS

- ¼ cup raw almonds
- ¼ cup raw cashews
- ¼ cup raw walnut halves
- Sea salt or kosher salt
- ¼ cup golden raisins
- ¼ cup dried cranberries
- ¼ cup dried apricots
- ¼ cup banana chips

DIRECTIONS

1. Preheat the oven to 350°. Spread the nuts on a baking sheet and toss with a pinch of salt. Toast for 10 minutes, stirring halfway through, until brown. Let the nuts cool completely. Mix the nuts with the dried fruits.

NUTRITIONAL INFORMATION

calories:200 Cal, carbohydrates:26g, protein:4g, Fats:9g, fiber:3g, sugar:20g, cholesterol:0mg

Roasted Chickpeas

- Prep time: 5 minutes
- Cook time: 20 minutes
- Total time: 25 minutes
- Serving:11/2 cups

INGREDIENTS

- 1 1/2 cups cooked chickpeas, drained and rinsed
- Extra-virgin olive oil, for drizzling
- Sea salt
- Paprika, curry powder, or other spices (optional)

DIRECTION

1. Preheat the oven to 425°F and lay parchment paper on a large baking sheet.

2. To dry, spread out the chickpeas on a kitchen towel. Remove any stray skins.

3. Toss the dry chickpeas with a drizzle of olive oil and liberal pinches of salt on a baking sheet.

4.   Cook the chickpeas for 20 to 30 minutes, or until golden brown and crispy. Ovens vary; if your chickpeas aren't crispy enough, continue cooking until they are!

5.   Remove from the oven and stir with pinches of your preferred spices, if using, while the chickpeas are still warm.

6.   Roasted chickpeas should be stored at room temperature in a loosely covered container. They are best used within two days.

NUTRITIONAL INFORMATION

calories: 115 Kcal, carbohydrates:12g, protein:6g, fats:3g, fiber:5g, sugar: 0.4g, salt: 0g

CHAPTER 10: DRINKS RECIPE

Green Tea

- Prep time:10 minutes
- Cook time:10 minutes
- Total: 20 minutes
- Serving:1 serving

INGREDIENTS

- 2 teaspoon green tea powder
- 2 cup water
- **TEA BAG VERSION:**
    - 1 cup water
    - 1 teaspoon honey
    - 1 no tea bag

DIRECTION

1. Add 2 cups water to a sauce pan.

2. Let it come to a rolling boil. Switch off.

3. Add 2 teaspoon tea leaves to it.

4. Give a quick mix.

5. Let it rest for 2 mins.

6. Strain the tea leaves.

7. Green Tea is ready!

8. Pour into serving glass and Serve!

For Tea bag version :

- First add 1 cup boiled water to a serving cup.
- Add the tea bag to it.
- Dip dip dip until the color changes.
- Now green tea is ready to serve!
- Add honey or sugar as per your preference. This is optional.
- Add 1/2 to 1 teaspoon honey to tea.

- Mix it well.

- Green tea is ready to serve!

NUTRITIONAL INFORMATION

calories: 22 Kcal, carbohydrates:6g, protein:0.1g, fats: 0.1g, fiber: 0.3g, sugar:5g

Raspberry leaf tea

- Prep time: 5 minutes ,
- total time: 5 minutes

INGREDIENTS

- For Fresh Tea: 7-10 fresh Wild Raspberry leaves.
- For Dried Tea: 1 tsp of dried Raspberry leaves and 2-3 dried Raspberries.

DIRECTION

For fresh Tea:

1. Making Raspberry Leaf tea is simple, Just steep 7-10 young, fresh raspberry leaves in

boiling water for 5 minutes and add sugar to taste if desired.

For Dried Tea:

1. Harvest and wash a desired amount of Raspberry leaves and Berries.
2. Dry the plants and berries in a dehydrator. Be aware that the berries will take a lot longer to dry due to their water content.
3. Store the leaves and berries in a clean, dry jar.
4. Use 1 tsp in a tea strainer and steep in just-boiled water for 5 minutes. The berries can be added straight into the cup. Add sugar to taste, if desired.

NUTRITIONAL INFORMATION

calories:6g, carbohydrates:1g, protein:0g, fats:0.1g, fiber:0g, sugar;0g

Beetroot And Carrot Juice

- Prep time:10 minutes
- Serving: 1 serving

INGREDIENTS:

- 2 medium-sized carrots
- 1 medium-sized beetroot
- 1-inch piece of ginger
- 1-2 tablespoons of honey (optional for sweetness)
- Water (as needed)

DIRECTION

1. Wash and peel the carrots and beetroot. Cut them into small pieces for easier blending.

2. Peel the ginger and chop it into smaller chunks.

3. In a blender or juicer, add the carrot, beetroot and ginger pieces.

4. Blend or juice the ingredients until smooth. If using a blender, you may need to add some water to achieve a liquid consistency.

5. Taste the juice and add honey if you prefer a sweeter taste. Honey is optional and can be omitted if you prefer the natural flavor of the vegetables.

6. Once the juice is well blended and sweetened to your liking, strain it through a fine-mesh strainer or a nut milk bag to remove any pulp and fiber.

7. Pour the freshly prepared carrot beetroot juice into a glass and it's ready to be served!

8. For the best taste and nutrition, consume the juice immediately. If you prefer it chilled,

you can refrigerate it for a short while before serving.

NUTRITIONAL INFORMATION

calories: 42 Kcal, carbohydrates: 9.7g, protein: 0.84g, sugar:6.33g, fiber:0.4g

Bone Broth

- Prep time:12 hours
- total time: 12 hours
- serving: 8 servings

INGREDIENTS

- Bones and carcass of 1 chicken (we suggest starting with a whole roasted chicken)
- 12 cups filtered water
- 2 Tbsp apple cider vinegar
- 1 generous pinch each sea salt and black pepper (plus more to taste)
- Rosemary/herbs (leftover from roasting chicken // optional)
- 1 sliced lemon (leftover from roasting chicken // optional)

DIRECTION

1. To a large pot or Dutch oven, add the bones leftover from a whole roasted chicken (including legs and wings that may have been on the serving platter), or the bones from 1 chicken purchased from a butcher. (Note: This can also be done in a Crock-Pot or Instant Pot.)

2. We also like adding the lemon wedges and rosemary that were cooked with our whole roasted chicken (optional).

3. Top with filtered water until generously covered (about 12 cups / 2880 ml). This should reduce down by about 1/3 or 1/2, leaving you with 6-8 cups of bone broth.

4. Next, add in a bit of salt and pepper to season the broth (you can add more later to taste).

5. Then add apple cider vinegar, which is added primarily because the acidity breaks down the

collagen and makes it more abundant in the broth. You can also sub lemon juice, but we prefer apple cider vinegar.

6. Bring to a boil, then reduce to a simmer and cover. Cook for at least 10-12 hours, or until reduced by 1/3 to 1/2. The more it reduces, the more intense the flavor will become and the more collagen will be extracted. We find 12 hours to be about right.

7. Strain and discard the bones. Either use immediately or store in glass jars and freeze up to 1-2 months or more. Just be sure to leave a couple inches at the top of the jar to allow for expansion in the freezer.

NUTRITIONAL INFORMATION

Serving: 1 cupCalories: 53 Kcal Carbohydrates: 0.9g
Protein: 5.3 g Fat: 2.9g Cholesterol: 2.63 mg
Fiber: 0 g Sugar: 0.4gq

Watermelon Smoothie With Mint

- Prep time: 10 minutes
- Total: 10 minutes
- Serving: 1 serving

INGREDIENTS

- 2 cups chopped seedless watermelon
- 1 cup peeled and seeded cucumber, chopped
- 3 large leaves fresh mint

DIRECTION

1. Place the diced watermelon and cucumber in a covered container and freeze for at least an hour before using. You may also omit this step and just add ice cubes to the blender.

2. Combine the watermelon, cucumber, and mint in a blender. Add a splash of filtered water then blend. To assist the ingredients

blend together, add a dash of water at a time as needed. Blend until smooth. Serve cold and enjoy!

NUTRITIONAL INFORMATION

calories: 107 kcal, carbohydrates: 26g, protein: 3g, fat: 1g, fiber: 2g, sugar:21g,

Golden Milk with Turmeric and Ginger

- Prep time: 5 minutes
- Cook time: 5 minute
- Total: 10 minutes
- Serving:2 serving

INGREDIENTS

- **1** stick cinnamon or 1/4 teaspoon ground cinnamon more as garnish at the end 2 inches fresh turmeric cut or 12 teaspoon ground turmeric spice 1 inch fresh ginger sliced or 12 teaspoon ground ginger
- 1/2 teaspoon coconut oil
- Pinch black pepper
- 1 tbsp maple syrup or honey, plus more to taste

DIRECTION

1. In a small saucepan, combine the milk, cinnamon stick, turmeric, ginger, coconut oil, and black pepper.
2. Cook, stirring often, until the mixture is heated but not boiling.
3. Give it a taste and add in your sweetener.
4. Strain it into your cups if you used fresh turmeric and ginger. If not, split it evenly between two cups.
5. If preferred, sprinkle with ground cinnamon. Serve

NUTRITIONAL INFORMATION

Calories: 147 kcal | Carbohydrates: 12g | Protein: 2g|
Fat: 11g Fiber: 2g Sugar:6g |

Kefir

- Prep time: 10 minutes
- Plus 18-24 hrs for fermenting

INGREDIENTS

- ½ tsp kefir grains
- 1 pint milk (organic whole milk for best results)
- 1 slice lemon or 1 drop lemon oil (optional)

You will also need

- 500ml clip-top jar with fermentation gasket (or jar, cover, and rubber band)
- a sieve, jug/bowl, storage bottle, or straining funnel, as well as a wide-necked bottle

DIRECTION

1. Put ½ tsp kefir grains in the jar. Fill the jar with milk, allowing around 2cm head space if using a clip top jar, or at least 5cm if using a cloth-covered jar.

2. Set aside for 18-24 hours at room temperature to ferment. When the milk thickens, it is fermented into kefir. It is usual for it to have hardened and divided, with pockets of whey developing.

3. If you can't strain it right away, put it in the fridge to keep it from fermenting more; the flavor can get rather strong; strain it anytime during the following 48 hours

4. Strain the kefir into the jug or container using a sieve or straining funnel. The grains are fairly hardy and can endure little churning.

5. You may drink it immediately, flavor it and chill it (a piece of lemon peel or a dab of

lemon oil adds a lovely fresh taste), or Allow it to sit at room temperature for a few hours to enhance the flavor. Refrigerating it will slow down the fermentation by the bacteria, and it should be usable for 7-10 days.

6. To produce additional kefir, rinse out the container, return the grains (no need to wash them), and begin again from the beginning.

NUTRITIONAL INFORMATION

calories: 63 Kcal, carbohydrates:4g, protein:3g, Fats:4g, salt:0.1g, sugar:4g, fiber:0g, saturates: 2g

Pomegranate Juice

- Prep time: 30 minutes
- Cook time: 1 minutes
- Total time: 31 minutes
- Serving:2 servings

INGREDIENTS

- 2 cups pomegranate seeds
- 2 cups still water/seltzer water divided
- ¼ teaspoon salt
- 2 teaspoons sugar optional

DIRECTION

1. Add pomegranate seeds with 1 cup water to the blender. Pulse for 5-10 seconds, or until the juice begins to separate

2. from the seeds. If you pulse for too long, the seeds will begin to break down.

3. Using a sieve, filter the juice. Gently press the seeds with the back of a spoon to separate the liquid from the seeds.

4. Add more water as per taste (or seltzer water) to the strained juice. Add a pinch of salt and sugar. Mix well. Serve chilled.

NUTRITIONAL INFORMATION

Calories: 151 kcal | Carbohydrates: 34g | Protein: 2g | Fat: 1g Fiber: 6g| Sugar: 26g

Tart Cherry Juice

- Prep time: 5 minutes.
- Cook time: 30 minutes
- serving: 24 servings

INGREDIENTS

- 4 lb tart cherries
- 8 cups water
- 2 lb sugar

DIRECTION

1. Wash and rinse the tart cherries, remove the stems but leave the pits, and bring the water and cherries to a boil in a large saucepan.
2. Simmer for 20 minutes.

3. Press the fruit to release extra juice through a fine mesh strainer.

4. Return the drained liquid to the saucepan and stir in the sugar. Simmer for 10 minutes, or until the sugar (or sweetener) has dissolved.

5. Pour into hot bottles and close. Boil in a canning pot with a rack on the bottom for 10 minutes.

NUTRITION INFORMATION

Calories: 4654, Fat: 4g, Saturated Fat: 1g, Carbohydrates: 1197g, Fiber: 38g, Sugar: 1138g, Protein: 19g

Matcha Smoothie with Almond Milk and Banana

- Prep time: 5 minutes.
- Cook time: 3 minutes.
- Additional time: 3 minutes
- total time: 11 minutes
- serving: 1 serving

INGREDIENTS

- 1 teaspoon matcha green tea powder
- 1 large banana
- One cup of soy, almond, or milk
- 1/2 cup ice cubes

DIRECTION

1. In a blender, puree each ingredient until it's smooth.

NUTRITIONAL INFORMATION

CALORIES: 177 Cal   TOTAL FAT: 5g. CHOLESTEROL: 10mg. 26g CARBOHYDRATES, 2g FIBER, 11g SUGAR, 9g PROTEIN

GrapeFruit Juice

- Prep time:5 minutes,
- total time: 5 minutes.
- Serving: 2 serving

INGREDIENTS

- 25 oz grapefruits, 2 medium; if feasible, choose pink or Star Ruby grapefruits
- 12 oz orange 1 medium; grapefruit orange juice optional.
- This will yield about 1 ¾ cups/420ml of juice

DIRECTION

With a Juicer

1. Peel the fruit.

2. Cut it into tiny pieces to suit the juicer chute.

3. Feed the grapefruit pieces through your juicer – and voila!

With a Blender

1. Peel and firmly slice the fruit into numerous pieces. Remove any remaining seeds with a fork.

2. Along with the fruit, add 1/4-1/2 cup of water (per fruit) to the machine.

3. Use coconut water or any other sort of juice (orange, apple, pineapple) to add taste.

4. Blend into a juicy, pulpy consistency. This will take between 45-60 seconds.

5. Pout the juice into your glass through a strainer or a nut milk bag/ muslin cloth for smoothness. Squeeze lightly if doing the latter, or you'll make a mess.

Using a Citrus Juicer or a Handheld Juicer

1. Start by slicing the grapefruit/s in half.

2. I recommend rubbing it against the counter for 20-30 seconds to loosen the liquid (and/or microwave it for 15-20 seconds) to get the most juice.

3. Some hand juicers just need pressing, and others require you to manually squeeze and rotate the fruit over the juicing element. Make sure to place a bowl underneath.

4. If you like pulp (for fiber) in your juice, you may add it directly from the remaining fruit..

NUTRITIONAL INFORMATION

Calories: 229kcal | Carbohydrates: 58g | Protein: 4g | Fat: 1g | Fiber: 10g | Sugar: 40g |

Mango Smoothie with Yogurt

- Prep time: 10 minutes.

- Cook time: 0 minutes.

- Total: 10 minutes

- serving: 2 servings

INGREDIENTS

- 1 cup peeled diced mango
- 1 cup nonfat plain yogurt or vanilla yogurt
- 1/2 cup crushed ice
- Milk, or water, optional

DIRECTION

1. Gather the ingredients.
2. In a blender, combine the chopped mango, yogurt, and ice.

3. Blend or process until smooth.

4. If the smoothie is too thick, add a splash of milk or water and re-blend.

5. Serve immediately. Enjoy.

NUTRITIONAL INFORMATION

Calories:113Kcal, Total Fat 1g,Total Carbohydrate:21g, Dietary Fiber 1g, Total Sugars 20g,Protein 7g,Cholesterol

Acai Bowls

- **Prep time:10 minutes,**
- total: 10 minutes.
- serving: 2-3 servings

INGREDIENTS

- Add to a high powered blender:
- 1 packet (100 grams) frozen acai berry packet
- 1/2 cup 100% apple juice from concentrate
- 1 small frozen banana
- 1/2 cup frozen strawberries
- 1/2 cup frozen blueberries
- **Toppings for your bowl:** (Below are my ideas; add your preferred toppings and add to your desired quantity. These topping ideas are for a single acai bowl.)

- 1 tablespoon honey (I prefer adding this to the mixture before pouring it on top)
- Handful granola
- Fresh strawberries, raspberries, blueberries, and bananas: thinly sliced or chopped fruit
- 1 tablespoon chia seeds
- 1-2 tablespoons coconut

DIRECTION

1. In a high-powered blender, combine the acai berry package, apple juice, banana, strawberries, and blueberries. Blend until smooth. Pour into a large bowl.

2. Top the bowl with your favorite toppings, such as granola, fresh (thinly sliced) fruit, chia seeds, and coconut! I recommend putting a spoonful of honey on top of everything. Enjoy immediately

NUTRITIONAL INFORMATION

Calories: 211 Kcal, Fat: 6g, Protein: 3g Carbs: 3g, Sugar: 19g, Fiber: 7g

Avocado Smoothie with Almond Milk

- Prep time: 10 minutes
- total time: 10 minutes.
- Serving: 1 serving

INGREDIENTS

- 1 ¼ cups almond milk
- 1 avocado - peeled, pitted, and sliced
- 1 small banana, sliced
- ¼ cup ice, or as needed
- 1 tablespoon honey (Optional)

DIRECTIONS

1. Blend almond milk, avocado, banana, ice, and honey in a blender until smooth.

NUTRITIONAL INFORMATION

Calories:555 Kcal, carbohydrates:68g, protein:7g, fats:33g, Dietary Fiber 18g,Total Sugars 40g

Orange Juice

- Cook time: 5 minutes.
- Total time:5 minutes.
- Serving: 2 servings

INGREDIENTS

- 2.5 pound oranges common, navel, Valencia, tangerines, clementines, satsuma, blood orange, etc.

DIRECTION

With A Juicer

1. Prepare the oranges by first peeling them. Then, cut them into smaller pieces to fit into your juicer tube.
2. Feed a few at a time into your juicer chute and voilà!

With A Blender

1. Peel the oranges and, if desired, remove and discard the seeds (if straining the juice, this isn't essential).

2. .Add the orange segments to a blender. If required, add a splash of water to help them mix (1/4 cup should be plenty to avoid over-watering).

3. Blend into a juicy, pulp consistency. Then strain the resultant pulpy juice through a sieve or nut milk bag, or leave it as is if you prefer orange juice with pulp (for extra nutrients).

With A Handheld Juice

1. This probably doesn't require much explanation. If you have a lemon/orange juicer, cut the fruit in half and set it over the juicer, pressing down and squeezing while

spinning back and forth to extract as much juice as possible.

2.   For orange juice with pulp, just spoon some directly out from the remaining orange (after squeezing the juice out) and add to your glass.

What to do with any leftover pulp

- Orange pulp can also be frozen into an ice-cube tray for later usage- within smoothies, broths, or baked goods. Alternatively, the pulp can be composted

NUTRITIONAL INFORMATION

Serving: 1 Cup | Calories: 266 kcal | Carbohydrates: 67g | Protein: 5g | Fat: 1g |Fiber: 14g | Sugar: 53g

CONCLUSION

How about we sum up the significant bits of knowledge that will go about as directing lights on your course to nurturing as we wrap up this journey into the domain of fruitfulness centered eating.

We've checked out the central connection among diet and fruitfulness on these pages, noticing that each significant piece adds to the confounded dance of contraceptive wellbeing. The dishes introduced here are more than basically culinary enjoyments; they are solicitations to embrace the groundbreaking capability of supplement rich, ripeness agreeable feasts.

Recollect that powering your body is an extensive movement as you start on your contraceptive excursion. The utilization of vivid foods grown from the ground, as well as lean proteins and complete grains, goes about as a reason for good regenerative wellbeing. The cautious choice of fixings, the equilibrium of supplements, and the delight of enjoying each chomp are fundamental parts of this connoisseur and invigorating experience.

Each little decision includes in the area of ripeness, and your way is remarkable to you. Acknowledge it with the mindfulness that you have command over your own prosperity. The desire to proceed plagues these pages — each step you take, each nutritious feast you eat, is a stage toward the future you need.

Therefore, my reader remains committed to this shifting course. Permit these dishes to enliven your table, yet in addition to give your body the nourishment it requires. May the kitchen become a safe-haven where you sustain your body as well as your yearnings of kids as you get familiar with the expertise of fruitfulness centered cooking.

At long last, recollect that your contraceptive excursion is a story that is developing with each conscious decision. The food you supply today lays the preparation for the sections to come. Your commitment to eating in a way that prioritizes fertility demonstrates your strength.

I wish you a prosperous excursion loaded with wellbeing, good faith, and the pleasure of gastronomic experience. May these recipes keep on being a wellspring of motivation and certainty for you as you navigate the exquisite excursion toward Life as a parent.

REVIEW

Dear Readers

I hope this communication finds you in good health.I trust you've had the valuable chance to dig into the pages of The Essential Fertility food cookbook and investigate the universe of fruitfulness centered sustenance.

As a creator committed to giving significant bits of knowledge and backing on the excursion to being a parent, I'm anxious to hear your considerations. Your criticism is massively significant and assumes a urgent part in molding the fate of my work.

In the event that you could save a couple of seconds to share your review, it would be profoundly valued. Your sincere opinions have the potential to have a significant impact on and serve as a guide for those who are navigating their own paths to parenthood.

Go ahead and feature angles you saw as especially supportive, any recipes you appreciated, or ideas for development. Your feedback will add to making content that resounds with and upholds people on their fruitfulness processes.

Much obliged to you for being important for this local area and for thinking about sharing your contemplations. Your help means everything.

Warm Regards,

Peggy M. Tharp

Author of The Essential Fertility Food cookbook

www.ingramcontent.com/pod-product-compliance
Lightning Source LLC
Chambersburg PA
CBHW070920260726
48661CB00003B/767